Managing Stress

From Morning to Night

Fitness, Health & Nutrition was created by Rebus, Inc. and published by Time-Life Books.

REBUS, INC.

Publisher: RODNEY FRIEDMAN

Editor: CHARLES L. MEE JR.
Executive Editor: THOMAS DICKEY
Managing Editor: SUSAN BRONSON
Senior Editor: WILLIAM DUNNETT
Associate Editors: MARY CROWLEY, CARL LOWE
Contributing Editors: MICHAEL GOLDMAN, PAUL PERRY

Art Director: JUDITH HENRY
Designer: DEBORAH RAGASTO
Photographer: STEVEN MAYS
Photo Stylist: NOLA LOPEZ

Recipe Editor: BONNIE J. SLOTNICK
Contributing Editor: MARYA DALRYMPLE
Test Kitchen Director: GRACE YOUNG
Nutritional Analyst: HILL NUTRITION ASSOCIATES

Chief of Research: CARNEY MIMMS
Assistant Editor: JACQUELINE DILLON

TIME-LIFE BOOKS

European Editor: Kit van Tulleken
Assistant European Editor: Gillian Moore
Design Director: Ed Skyner
Chief of Research: Vanessa Kramer
Chief Sub-Editor: Ilse Gray

EUROPEAN EDITION

Designer: Paul Reeves
Sub-Editor: Douglas Amrine
Chief of Editorial Production: Maureen Kelly
Production Assistant: Deborah Fulham
Editorial Department: Theresa John, Debra Lelliott

FITNESS, HEALTH & NUTRITION

Managing Stress
From Morning to Night

TIME
LIFE
BOOKS

Time-Life Books, Amsterdam

CONSULTANTS FOR THIS BOOK

Herbert Benson, M.D., is Associate Professor of Medicine at the Harvard Medical School, Massachusetts. He is the author of *The Relaxation Response* and *The Maximum Mind*.

Ann Grandjean, M.S., is chief nutrition consultant to the U.S. Olympic Committee and an instructor in the Sports Medicine Program, University of Nebraska Medical Center.

Kenneth R. Pelletier, Ph.D., M.D., is Associate Clinical Professor in the Department of Medicine and the Department of Psychiatry, University of California School of Medicine, San Francisco. He has written more than 150 articles on behavioural medicine, clinical feedback and neurophysiology.

Paul J. Rosch, M.D., is President of the American Institute of Stress and Clinical Professor of Medicine and Psychiatry, New York Medical College. He is also a Fellow of the Royal Society of Medicine and a Fellow of the World Academy of Art and Science.

John White, Ph.D., is Reader in Human Sciences at the West London Institute of Higher Education, with responsibilities for undergraduate teaching and postgraduate research in exercise physiology.

Myron Winick, M.D., is Professor of Nutrition at Columbia University College of Physicians and Surgeons, New York.

The following consultants helped design the exercise sequences in this book:

Kevin Gardiner conducts classes in Yoga and Tai Chi in New York.

Charlotte Honda has been a dance and movement teacher for 25 years. She currently teaches Hatha Yoga and modern dance in New York.

Nancy Klitsner, who holds a master's degree in applied physiology, is an exercise physiologist in private practice in New York.

Paul McGregor is a graduate of the Swedish Institute of Massage and a licensed massage therapist.

CONTENTS

CHAPTER ONE

Recognizing Stress

The sources, the effects, the warning signals — and the benefits of coping

S tress is inescapable, reaching into your work environment, social affairs and home life, and even intruding on your sleep. Stress-related problems have become an ever-increasing complaint among people who work, from those on an assembly line to top-level executives, and symptoms linked to stress account for a high proportion of all visits to family doctors.

Many people think of stress only as a negative force, sapping their energy and decision-making abilities, decreasing their productivity and making them more susceptible to illness. Yet researchers have shown that stress can also have a positive side, and that in fact some stress is necessary for functioning effectively and living a full life. Whether stress has a mostly positive or negative impact on you depends on how you perceive and respond to stressful situations. And recognizing stress and then coping with it successfully are processes that you can learn.

7

Sources of Stress

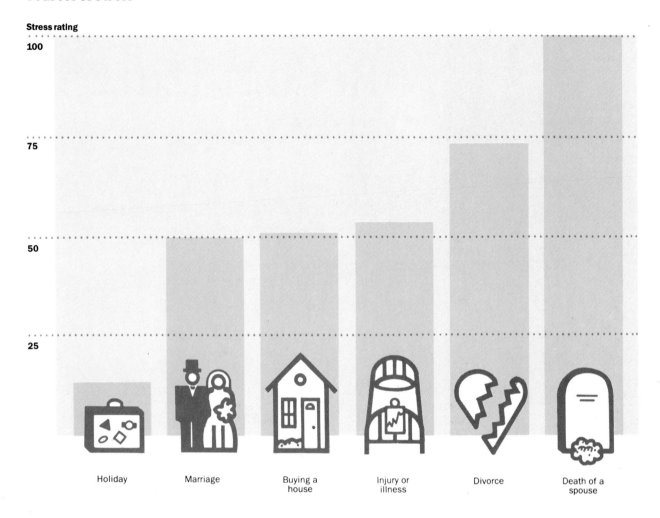

Stress rating

100

75

50

25

Holiday　　Marriage　　Buying a house　　Injury or illness　　Divorce　　Death of a spouse

Change is stressful, whether it is a happy or unhappy change. This is what stress researchers Thomas Holmes and Richard Rahe found during the 1960s, when they studied the reactions of more than 5,000 subjects to events in their lives. Holmes and Rahe found that the event consistently reported as more stressful than all others was the death of a spouse. They assigned bereavement a value of 100 and they devised a Social Readjustment Rating Scale that compared other life events to it, as shown in this chart.

What is stress?

There is no simple definition of stress: the term has been used by researchers and the public alike to refer to both the effects of stress and the stressors, which are events or conditions that produce stress. In general, though, stress can be thought of as the perception that events or circumstances have challenged, or exceeded, a person's ability to cope. This emphasizes the lesson that stress researchers have learned repeatedly, which is that stress occurs within each individual and is determined by his or her particular characteristics. This helps explain why some events — a deadline at work, for example — can almost paralyse one person but inspire another.

Since the responses to stressors vary so greatly, researchers often classify them according to the time span in which they occur. Thus, stressors can be immediate and short term, such as waiting for a job interview; they can be protracted and chronic, such as a family conflict or a noisy environment; or they can be events that trigger a series of major life changes, such as being sacked or getting a divorce.

Our reactions to stressors can be divided into two broad categories: psychological and physiological. On the psychological level, we often respond to stressors unpredictably, as variations in our moods and emotions trigger changes in our behaviour, ranging from expressions of anger to patterns of alcohol or drug use. Your psychological reaction to a stressor depends on many factors, including your emotional state at the time and how troublesome you perceive the stressor to be.

Your physiological response to stress, shown in the illustration on page 12 called "The Biochemistry of Stress", is more predictable than the psychological response. A stressor sets in motion a series of bio-chemical and neurological changes that is much the same regardless of the stressor that provoked it.

Is stress always negative?

Not at all. A number of studies have shown that some degree of stress is important for human development. As early as 1908, two researchers at Harvard University discovered that, up to a point, increased stress results in improved performance and efficiency — a principle illustrated in the bell curve on page 24. At certain times and under certain conditions, stress helps to improve your self-esteem and competence, enhance your personal development and relieve boredom. In many activities, you may need some level of stress to perform well and to meet new challenges. An area in which stress has been shown most clearly to help performance is athletics. In one American study of children's baseball leagues, researchers looked at how the stress of being up at bat related to performance. Batters who showed either high or low levels of anxiety did not perform as well as batters who displayed a moderate amount of stress. Too little stress, in other words, can be as detrimental as too much.

Are some people addicted to stress?

Laboratory experiments show that animals exposed to stress have high levels of stress hormones, including opioid peptides, which closely resemble morphine in their chemical structure and effect. Humans, too, produce opioid peptides, leading some researchers to conclude that it is possible for people to become "addicted" to their own morphine-like stress hormones.

One researcher has even postulated the existence of a Type T personality, who tends to seek thrills, excitement, stimulation or arousal in high-risk activities. A positive Type T personality will take risks in such activities as hang gliding, scuba diving and rock climbing, whereas a negative Type T personality finds pleasure in crime, violence or driving while intoxicated.

Positive Type T personalities, however, show few characteristics that may be regarded as "addictive". According to a personality study of 293 high-risk competitors, including racing-car drivers, parachutists and aerobatic pilots, the subjects tended to be extremely successorientated, strongly extroverted and above average in intelligence and abstract reasoning ability. Further, they tended to be cool and calculating in their risk-taking.

What are the biggest sources of stress?

One major attempt to measure the degree of stress a situation or event produces was undertaken in the 1960s by Thomas Holmes, M.D., a psychiatrist at the University of Washington's School of Medicine, and a colleague, psychologist Richard Rahe. Working with tuberculosis patients and U.S. Navy ratings, Holmes and Rahe found that people who reported the most changes in their lives — either positive or negative — also seemed to suffer the most illnesses.

Combining their results, Holmes and Rahe devised a 100-point scale that rated 43 life events (later revised to 63) based on their estimated impact as stressors — that is, on the comparative severity and duration of the readjustment these changes demanded. Called the Social Readjustment Rating Scale, it set the death of a spouse at the top (100 points), followed by divorce (73), marital separation (65) and a prison sentence (63); at the lower end of the scale were such items as applying for a small loan (17), going on holiday (13) and getting booked for a traffic offence (11). Over the past 20 years, the Holmes-Rahe rating scale has been tested on thousands of people of many ages, races and cultures round the world, and the results have shown a surprising degree of consistency.

What about the effect of minor but more frequent stressors?

While the Holmes-Rahe scale is valuable for assessing the stress of major life changes, more recent research conducted by Richard Lazarus, M.D., and a group of his colleagues at the University of California at Berkeley indicates that relatively unimportant events — what the researchers characterize as "hassles" — have an even greater impact on your well-being.

Hassles range from getting stuck in a traffic jam to becoming involved in a dispute at work or misplacing your address book. The stress of a given hassle depends on a variety of factors: your style of coping, your personality and what the rest of your day was like, as well as the nature of the hassle itself. But the real effect of hassles is cumulative: unlike the stressful effects of major events, which are often isolated from one another and may be cushioned by the passage of time, hassles are constant, everyday stressors that become chronic and therefore have a long-term effect. Hassles, Dr. Lazarus found, have an impact on emotions and health. This is not to deny the impact of major setbacks. But Dr. Lazarus' findings suggest that the greatest stress of major events can often come from the daily disruptions they provoke. Besides the stressful blow to self-esteem of getting sacked, for example, there are the financial and personal hassles which are often associated with being out of work.

Does watching television relax you at the end of a hard day? On a regular basis, probably not. An American study indicates that heavy television watchers — both children and adults — overestimate the amount of violence in the real world, believe that policemen are routinely violent, and tend to mistrust others and to view themselves as living in a hostile world. This outlook is hardly stress-relieving; in fact, it is characteristic of the cardiac-prone personality researchers have found to be the most vulnerable to stress.

Little Hassles, Big Stresses

Although most people assume that major upheavals such as the death of a spouse or the purchase of a house cause the greatest stress, a study at the University of California, Berkeley, indicates that everyday aggravations may take the greatest toll. Researchers found that the cumulative stress of such hassles as housework, irritating noise, too many responsibilities, constant interruptions and rising prices can far outweigh that of a major trauma.

Dr. Lazarus' research is encouraging in that it depicts stress as manageable. Although hassles are unavoidable occurrences in day-to-day living, they can often be modified or avoided more easily than many major life-changing events.

How does your body respond to stress?

Although the situations or events that elicit stress vary from one person to another, physiologists have long known that people undergo the same general response to stress. Imagine that you are quietly reading when a nearby fire alarm goes off by accident. You are frightened by the sudden sound, and you jump from your chair and wonder whether to call the fire brigade. Realizing that there is no emergency, you settle down and continue reading, trying to cope with the sound of loudly ringing bells. After a while, though, you become so annoyed and agitated that you cannot continue reading.

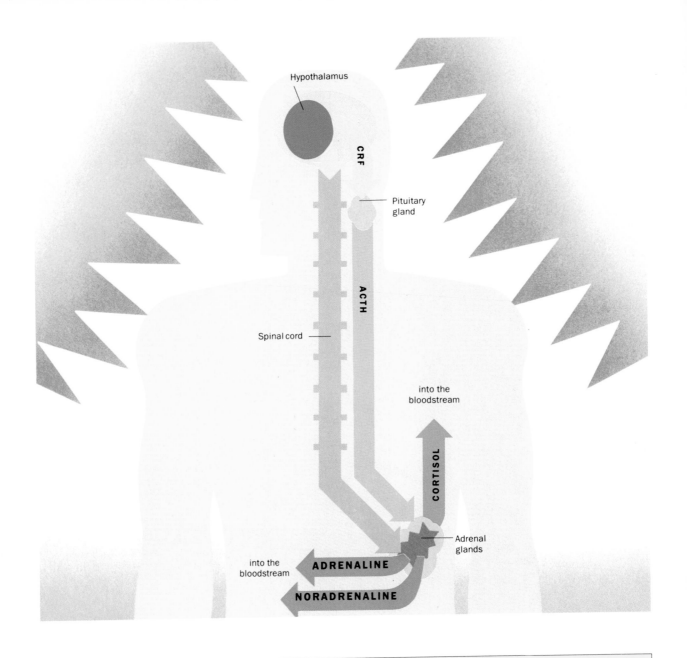

The Biochemistry of Stress

Virtually any stressful event, from quarrelling with a boss to winning a lottery, triggers an array of neural and biochemical reactions that prepares you to cope.

First, activity in the brain sparks the hypothalamus into action. As shown above, the hypothalamus secretes a substance called CRF, which sends messages down two pathways. On one track, nerve cells in the brain stem and spinal cord relay impulses to the core of the adrenal glands (located on top of the kidneys). These glands secrete adrenaline and noradrenaline, neurochemicals that prime the body for action by increasing heart rate, breathing, alertness and muscle response. This chain of neurological events is often called the fight-or-flight reaction.

Simultaneously, the CRF secreted by the hypothalamus causes the pituitary gland, located at the base of the brain, to produce ACTH, a hormone that tells the surface of the adrenal glands to release cortisol into the bloodstream. Cortisol sets off reactions that speed up the body's metabolism.

These two tracks feed back to the pituitary gland to regulate the stress response further. Although triggering this response may help you deal with stress, repeated exposure can damage you mentally and physically.

You react to the ringing bells in roughly the same way you would if you were to jump into a pool of cold water or be frightened by a large dog. This reaction is what Hans Selye, a pioneer in research into the physiology of stress, called the General Adaptation Syndrome. An Austrian scientist who emigrated to Canada in the 1930s, Selye believed that this syndrome is a response to almost any stressor. According to Selye, the syndrome occurs in three stages — alarm, resistance and exhaustion. The alarm stage produces changes in the brain and endocrine system. Perhaps the most dramatic and best known of these physiological responses is the group of reactions called the fight-or-flight response.

What is the fight-or-flight response?

Named by physiologist Walter B. Cannon at Harvard Medical School in the 1920s, the fight-or-flight response swings the body into physiological high gear in preparation to confront a threat, escape from it or try to repair injuries. The response is triggered by the sympathetic nervous system, which stimulates a discharge of the stress hormones adrenaline and noradrenaline from the adrenal glands. These two hormones prepare the body for action and help produce a wide range of changes in the body. The changes can include a near-shutdown of the digestive system and improved visual perception and muscle response, as well as higher blood pressure, bloodsugar and cholesterol levels, and increased breathing and heart rates.

What happens after fight-or-flight?

If a stressor persists for more than a brief time, the body adapts to it by entering the stage of resistance. During this phase the body's systems return to normal, but they remain alert to respond to the stressor. If the stressor is intense or long-lasting, the body eventually enters the third and final stage, exhaustion, at which point it is no longer able to resist the stressor. The body then becomes vulnerable to dysfunction and disease.

When you are in a threatening situation, the fight-or-flight response is clearly useful. It may also serve you when confronting a non-threatening challenge, as in an athletic competition or meeting a deadline at work. But in modern society, the fight-or-flight response is often provoked when it is neither needed nor useful — in an argument, for example, or while you are waiting in a long queue at the bank or at a supermarket checkout counter. Your body is in a heightened state, but it has no way to release its pent-up energy. And without alternative methods of coping with stress, stifling the alarm reaction can be physically and psychologically damaging.

How else does stress get out of hand?

In studying the effects of stress, researchers have determined that the impact of a stressor depends to a great extent on your perception of its frequency and duration. An acute stressor is immediate and identifiable, such as waiting to see a dentist or making an important speech. After you have finished dealing with this source of stress, you relax temporarily and then proceed to other tasks. As long as you can cope with each acute stressor as and when it arises, stress remains both short term and manageable.

Acutely stressful situations, however, can accumulate to cause long-term stress. A cluster of stressors may occur in such rapid succession that you do not have enough time to adapt — for example, a deadline is moved up at your office just as a valuable employee leaves. Or a stressor can be intermittent, occurring on a more or less regular basis that you have little control over, such as driving to work in rush-hour traffic. Finally, there are chronic stress conditions, which are the result of such constant stressors as a disabling illness or persistent tensions at home or at work.

What are some of the warning signals that an overload of stress is building up?

Signals that you are under too much stress range from general malaise to physical pain. These symptoms are so wide-ranging that people often do not recognize them as signs of stress. They include emotional responses such as overreacting to minor problems, inappropriate anger or impatience, overeating or loss of appetite, and increased use of alcohol, tobacco or drugs. If you are suffering from stress overload, you may feel anxious, be unable to relax or experience long periods of boredom. Too much stress can also disrupt sleeping patterns, sexual activity and performance at work.

Under stress, many people show a diminished ability to set priorities and make decisions. They attack tasks with less certainty and make more mistakes. In one study of university students, for example, researchers imposed high stress on subjects taking an examination. Not only did it take much longer for the students to complete the examination, but their error rate rose dramatically as well.

Finally, stress overload may manifest itself in physical symptoms, such as headaches, cold hands or feet, indigestion, aching neck or back, ulcers, nausea, diarrhoea or constipation, shortness of breath, heart palpitations, teeth grinding, muscle spasms and skin conditions such as acne and psoriasis. People under stress also lose more time from work because of illness.

Is there a direct relationship between stress overload and illness?

Stress has been implicated in various health breakdowns. According to Holmes and Rahe, people whose stressors add up to between 150 and 300 points on the Social Readjustment Rating Scale run a 50 per cent chance of falling seriously ill or being involved in a serious accident within about six months; if their score exceeds 300, the probability soars to 80 per cent. And one study further indicated that subjects with high

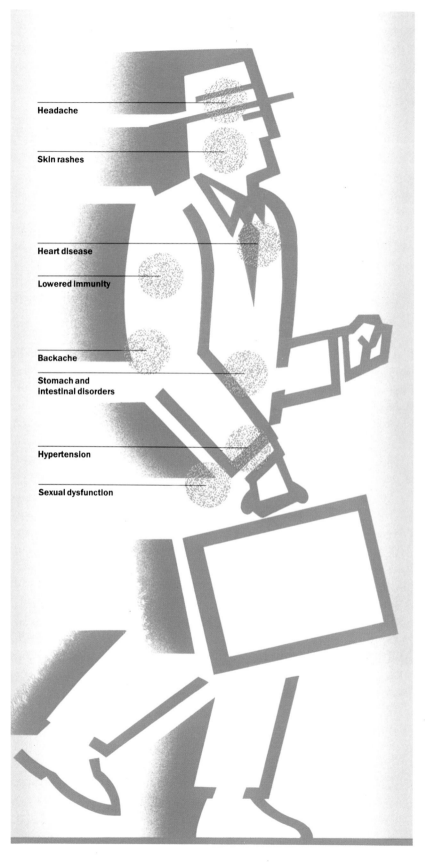

Headache

Skin rashes

Heart disease

Lowered immunity

Backache

Stomach and
intestinal disorders

Hypertension

Sexual dysfunction

The Physical Toll

Stress appears to influence a wide range of diseases and disorders. The most crucial response in this respect may be the suppression of the body's immune response. In one study, for example, during stressful examination periods, antibody levels in students were found to be lower than normal, indicating a greater vulnerability to infection. Other studies have shown that aggressive Type A personalities catch more colds than their more relaxed Type B counterparts.

Many studies have found a strong connection between heart disease and stress, especially in Type A personalities. Moreover, other studies have suggested a link between high cholesterol levels, a contributing factor in heart disease, and occupational stress.

Many ailments of the stomach and intestinal tract are strongly influenced by one's emotional state. Likewise, headaches and backaches have long been linked to stress. In one study comparing a headache-prone group with a headache-free group, the headache sufferers showed a significantly higher stress response following a test. And in another study, backache sufferers scored higher than healthy subjects on all measures of stress, including the Holmes-Rahe scale *(see illustration, page 8)*.

Stress also appears to be linked with many skin disorders. In a recent Swedish study, psoriasis sufferers showed higher levels of stress hormones than healthy subjects when subjected to stressful tests.

Evidence is accumulating that stress may pose a special threat to people with chronic hypertension. In one study, both hypertensive and borderline hypertensive subjects showed higher levels of stress hormones when given a word-matching test than did subjects with normal blood pressure.

Medical research has also begun to reveal the links between stress and sexual problems. In one study, for example, men who experienced the least arousal when viewing erotic films had the highest levels of the stress hormone cortisol.

Holmes-Rahe scores suffered not only serious illness or injury, but also such minor setbacks as colds and cuts and bruises.

In his study of day-to-day stress, Richard Lazarus at Berkeley found that hassles were an even better predictor of health problems than major life changes. The more frequent and intense the hassles that subjects reported, the greater their risk of high blood pressure, asthma attacks, chest pains and other complaints.

The extent to which stress causes illness has not been conclusively shown, since most studies deal only with people with existing medical complaints and are dependent on their often unreliable recall of past stressful events. But evidence that stress is a crucial factor in physical and emotional health continues to mount.

Are the health consequences of stress the same for both men and women?

According to a study of 311 male and 171 female executives, men and women responded to stress somewhat differently. Male executives with stress-related problems tended to suffer from physical illnesses, such as ulcers and cardiovascular disease, while women more often developed mental disorders, such as excessive anxiety, obsessions and depression. But men and women with stress-related illnesses also had many similarities — among them alcohol abuse, a sedentary lifestyle and compulsive work habits.

To what extent is stress responsible for heart attacks?

Although the biochemistry of stress is not fully understood, it is known that stress can raise your blood cholesterol level, which increases your risk of cardiovascular disease. In a study of accountants, researchers found that the subjects' cholesterol levels increased by 20 per cent during times of intense work pressure. Other research has clearly shown a direct correlation between high blood cholesterol levels and increased risk of cardiovascular disease and heart attack. And after more than two decades of studying the link between cardiovascular disease and personality, researchers assembled by the U.S. National Heart, Lung and Blood Institute determined that individuals who are in a daily tug of war with stress — Type A personalities — are at greater risk of developing cardiovascular disease than those who take a more relaxed approach to the stressors of daily life, or Type Bs. In fact, the Type A personality was found to predict coronary heart disease as effectively as such traditional risk factors as hypertension, high cholesterol levels and smoking did.

What is a Type A personality?

Cardiologist Meyer Friedman, M.D., director of the Recurrent Coronary Prevention Project in San Francisco, has identified traits and behaviour patterns typical of Type A personalities. According to Dr.

Friedman, Type A personalities tend to be excessively aggressive, competitive and ambitious. They are often insecure about their status and are therefore constantly trying to accomplish more and more. Dr. Friedman has also identified a "hurry sickness" in Type A personalities, a constant sense of urgency and a need to achieve too much in too little time. They frequently attempt to do many things at once; a Type A personality may consider simultaneously eating, reading and catching up on phone calls an efficient use of his lunch hour.

One component of the Type A personality that is particularly linked with heart attacks is hostility. Type A people who harbour free-floating hostility — usually expressed as excessive anger, annoyance or impatience — have been shown to have five to six times as many heart attacks as those who do not display this trait.

Type B personalities are usually described in the negative sense of simply not having Type A traits. Type B people do not have a constant sense of urgency. They can arrange a schedule that allows them to do one thing at a time. They can relax. They do not harbour a free-floating hostility; they can put themselves in other people's positions and appreciate their feelings. A sense of greater self-esteem is also a mark of Type B personalities; they are less likely than Type A people to try continually to prove themselves.

Most people, Friedman has pointed out, are not purely Type A or Type B, but exhibit characteristics of both types at different times. However, people who exhibit Type A behaviour much or all of the time have an 80 per cent greater risk of cardiovascular disease than those who are more consistently Type B. Curiously, heart-attack victims with Type A personalities are more likely to survive the episode than Type B personalities, a fact that researchers cannot yet explain.

Isn't it true that Type A personalities are generally more successful than Type Bs?
Western society does tend to reward aggressive people more than non-aggressive people. But it is by no means true that only Type A personalities can succeed. Some world leaders have been Type B personalities. In fact, based on interviews with more than 100 Nobel laureates and leaders in business, law, journalism, politics, education, religion and the military, Meyer Friedman and his associates found that only 65 per cent were Type A. Moreover, of the Type B corporate executives Dr. Friedman included in his survey, not one has suffered a heart attack before the age of 65.

Can people with Type A personalities modify their behaviour?
Although no reliable long-term study has yet confirmed this, many researchers believe that behavioural modification is not only possible but necessary for Type A people to reduce their risk of cardiovascular disease. First, Type A individuals must become aware of their behav-

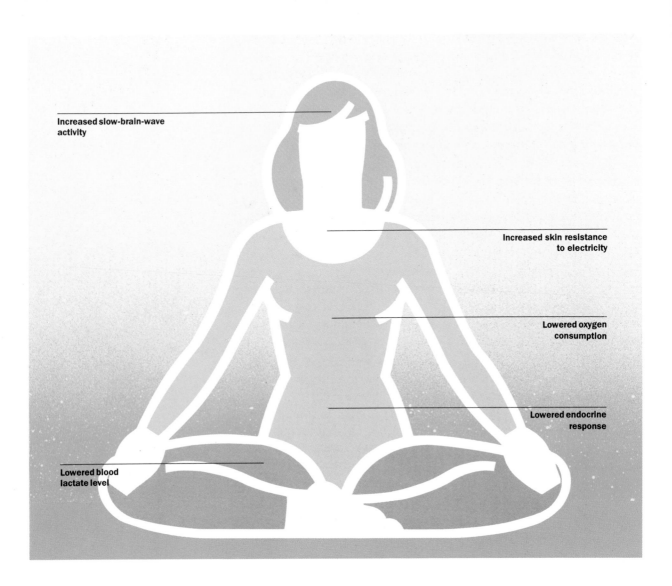

Increased slow-brain-wave
activity

Increased skin resistance
to electricity

Lowered oxygen
consumption

Lowered endocrine
response

Lowered blood
lactate level

The Relaxation Response

Just as stress triggers a set of biochemical responses, so does relaxation — in fact, it triggers nearly the opposite responses to stress. In a series of experiments at Harvard Medical School, researchers working with Herbert Benson, M.D., monitored subjects who used various meditation techniques to achieve a relaxed state. Dr. Benson called the changes produced by this state the relaxation response.

As this illustration shows, indications of basic physiological activity begin to decline as the body becomes relaxed. Heartbeat and breathing slow, oxygen consumption decreases and the level of blood lactate — a by-product of muscular activity associated with anxiety — falls rapidly. At the same time, the skin's resistance to electricity increases, a measurement that reveals lower levels of tension. People who are hypertensive also experience a decline in blood pressure.

Changes in the nervous and endocrine system are equally dramatic. The intensity of slow alpha waves in the brain increases, a change characteristic of relaxed wakefulness. And although the body continues to secrete stress hormones such as adrenaline, the body's response to them, as measured by blood pressure, is diminished.

For guidelines on how to invoke the relaxation response through meditation, see pages 52-53.

iour and of the circumstances that lead to their intense anxiety, frustration or anger. Once aware, they can modify either their behaviour or the circumstances that cause their stress. One way many Type A people can alter their behaviour is through time management. By pacing themselves so that they work on one task at a time, rather than constantly battling against the clock with an overload of activities, they can learn to become more relaxed and more productive.

How does stress make you more susceptible to disease?

Since ancient times, doctors have known that people who are under stress tend to develop illnesses more often than those who are not. But until recently, many scientists believed that the immune system operated independently of other physiological systems and psychological conditions. People exposed to viruses, they reasoned, were either immune or they became ill. Now, however, there is mounting evidence that stress increases vulnerability to infectious diseases. Researchers have discovered a link between stress and such illnesses as tuberculosis, glandular fever, streptococcal infections, herpes simplex, poliomyelitis and even the common cold. Certainly stress does not cause the infection — it takes a virus, fungus or bacterium to do that — but stress does reduce the body's resistance to such pathogens.

Researchers have conducted a number of studies showing that psychological events can influence immune-system functioning and, as a result of these findings, there is a new field called psychoneuroimmunology. In many studies in this area, researchers have measured significant depression of the immune system during times of intense stress, such as bereavement or anguish over a divorce. In one study comparing blood samples of women who had been divorced for one year or less to those who were still married, researchers found that the divorced women had depressed immunity. The less time that had passed since the divorce, the more impaired a woman's immune system was.

In addition, scientists have determined that even relatively commonplace stress can adversely affect the immune system. In one study, blood samples were taken from first-year medical students on two occasions — a month before final exams and again on the first day of exam week. Analysis of the blood samples revealed significant immune-system impairment at the time of the finals.

Has stress been implicated in causing cancer?

Important to the immune response of both animals and humans, natural killer cells seek out and destroy cancer cells. When natural killer cells are depressed, cancers can rapidly develop and spread to other parts of the body. A research study conducted with rats determined that uncontrollable stressors — for example, intermittent electric shocks — can reduce the effectiveness of natural killer cells.

S tudies have shown that stress can weaken the body's immune system. Now a recent study indicates that feelings of altruism may benefit the immune system. A group of college students viewed two films — one about Nazi Germany, the other about Mother Teresa's work with the poor in India. While they watched the Mother Teresa film, the students' feelings of friendliness and generosity rose, and their overall outlook became more positive. At the same time, their blood levels of immunoglobulin, which is made up of infection-fighting proteins, climbed. No such effects were observed when students watched the other film.

Obviously, such an experiment cannot be ethically conducted on humans. However, a study based on a questionnaire and blood samples taken by researchers at Harvard University Medical School found that people who reported many life stressors and who were depressed and anxious were most likely to have low natural killer cell activity. Other studies show that people under stress tend to have lower blood levels of infection-fighting T-lymphocytes.

Can managing stress improve immunity to disease?

Psychoneuroimmunologists believe that people who actively manage stress are less likely to develop infectious diseases and perhaps even cancer. In one experiment, two groups of rats were placed in boxes with wheels in them. Both groups received intermittent electrical shocks (or stressors) to their tails, but only one group could shut off the shock by turning the wheel. The duration of the shock to the rats in the uncontrollable-stressor group was determined by the duration of the shock to the controllable-stressor group. The researchers found that the immune systems of the animals in the controllable-stressor group responded to infection just as well as a control group that did not receive any shocks at all, while the immune systems in the uncontrollable-stressor group did not respond as effectively.

Studies on humans are more difficult to perform, but it appears that the way in which people handle stress has an important influence on their immune system. In the Harvard University study cited on page 19, researchers found that subjects who could deal with a large number of stressful events without becoming depressed and anxious had the highest blood levels of natural killer cells of all the test subjects — even higher than those who reported little stress.

What distinguishes people who manage stress successfully?

In an eight-year study, University of Chicago researchers examined how middle and upper-level managers coped with stress. Those who handled stress well, the researchers noted, shared three common personality traits: commitment, control and challenge. These executives did not feel alienated or bored by their work; rather, they approached their work enthusiastically and rarely gave up in the face of obstacles. Further, they felt that they could influence events at their company and even turn situations to their advantage. They rarely felt that they were passive victims caught by forces beyond their control. Finally, those who handled stress well viewed change as stimulating and useful, rather than threatening or disruptive.

Can smoking reduce stress?

Apparently it can. Smoking is one of a number of "quick fixes" people turn to for reducing stress (see chart, page 31), and behavioural scientists have long been puzzled by the stubborn persistence of cigarette smoking, even among individuals who wish to stop. Now

How Fitness Beats Stress

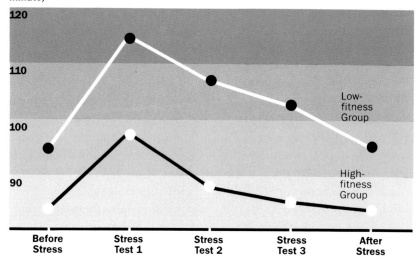

Pulse (beats per minute)

120
110
100
90

Low-fitness Group

High-fitness Group

Before Stress | Stress Test 1 | Stress Test 2 | Stress Test 3 | After Stress

This graph shows the results of a university study in which 10 highly fit students took a series of mildly stressful word-memory tests. Their pulse levels — recorded at each stage — were compared with those of less fit students given the same tests. Both groups of students showed the same levels of subjective emotional response to the tests. Their physiological responses to stress, however, were very different. Not only did the fitter students have lower pulse rates throughout, but their pulse rates also rose less after each test and declined more rapidly after the first test — demonstrating that the fitter students responded more calmly to the source of stress. (The pulses of all the students were somewhat higher than usual at the start of the test, probably due to the tension of an unfamiliar setting.)

it appears that smoking cigarettes is in many ways a "coping response" to the stress of daily living. Without cigarettes, many smokers feel unable to perform or compete.

No matter how stress-relieving smoking may be in the short term, though, its long-term effects are devastating. Smokers suffer significantly higher rates of hypertension, cardiovascular disease, respiratory illness, stroke and cancer. In addition, smoking markedly impairs the immune response to infectious diseases and cancer.

Does alcohol reduce stress effectively?

Research into the effects of alcohol on stress has produced mixed findings. While alcohol consumption by non-alcoholic drinkers generally results in elevated moods and reduced anxiety, most people drink to attain those benefits and therefore prejudice the results. In one study, one group of subjects was given the equivalent of two drinks of vodka, while another group was given an equal amount of tonic water and vitamin C. Half of the subjects in each group were told they were given alcohol, and the other half were told they were given vitamin C. Those who thought they had consumed alcohol — whether or not they actually did — reported greater mood elevation than those who thought they had consumed vitamin C. Expectation of mood change as a result of drinking alcohol, therefore, is apparently more powerful than the actual effect of the drink.

Can you laugh stress away?

American author Norman Cousins wrote a best-seller, *Anatomy of an Illness*, detailing how he recovered from a lingering and potentially

21

Stress may promote dental cavities. In an American study, stress caused subjects to produce saliva containing proteins involved in the formation of plaque, a bacterial coating that encourages cavities. But after 20 minutes of meditation, the same subjects had lower levels of plaque-forming bacteria in their mouths. Even more surprising, during relaxation the subjects' salivary glands produced saliva with high levels of calcium, phosphorus and fluoride — all of which protect tooth enamel.

fatal illness — ankylosing spondylitis. Paralysed and racked by pain, he watched Marx Brothers films and other comedies in his hospital room. To his delight, laughter seemed to induce pain-free sleep. Moreover, his sedimentation rate — a blood test used to measure the seriousness of infection — improved after each screening. According to Cousins, this proved the validity of the folk wisdom that laughter is the best medicine. He referred to it as "internal jogging".

At first, the medical community did not take Cousins' claims seriously. But subsequent research has shown that laughing can indeed be thought of as internal jogging: laughing increases respiratory exchange, heart rate, muscular activity and body temperature, and it stimulates the production of beta-endorphins, the chemicals some researchers believe are responsible for "runner's high". Recent studies at the University of California found that laughter was as effective in reducing stress as complex biofeedback training programmes. And laughter, the researchers noted, requires no special training or equipment — just a sense of humour.

Does crying reduce stress?

Chemical analysis of tears shed by people watching harrowing films compared to those of people exposed to onion vapours shows that the emotional tears contain significantly more protein. Tears, in theory, may help remove chemicals that build up during an emotionally stressful situation, thus restoring the body's chemical balance.

Whatever the chemical or physiological purpose of crying, it is an effective way of reducing psychological tension. In one survey, 73 per cent of the men and 85 per cent of the women questioned asserted that they felt better after crying. Another study compared a group of men and women with stress-related disorders to a group of healthy people of similar age and background. The researchers found that one difference between the two groups was that subjects who were ill tended to regard crying as a sign of weakness or loss of control, whereas members of the healthy group were not ashamed to cry. Another study showed that widows who wept and expressed their emotions when their husbands died were not as susceptible to stress-related illness as those who did not grieve openly.

Although crying will not remove the source of stress, it does aid relaxation and help to clear the mind so that we can begin again to cope with stressful events.

Is it possible to become immune to stress?

While it is certainly not possible to become totally immune to stress, you can become "inoculated" against stress to make it more bearable and to reduce its harmful effects. During World War II, for instance, recruits were battle-inoculated by listening to lectures and watching films about the realities of combat. Many were then subjected to simulated battle conditions. Battle inoculation helped to reduce soldiers' anxiety during actual combat, increase their self-confidence and improve their performance under extremely stressful conditions.

Mental or physical rehearsals of stress-inducing situations have more recently been used in a number of settings. Teenagers, for instance, can be protected against the stress of peer pressure to smoke cigarettes or take drugs by role-playing. By rehearsing how they will handle difficult confrontations, they can more effectively deal with the actual situation when it arises. Doctors often help patients become inoculated against the stress of surgery by carefully reviewing the surgical procedure beforehand, with all of its dangers, discomforts and ultimate benefits. Studies show that stress inoculation enables patients to deal better with the stress of unpleasant treatments and to recover more quickly.

Can your ties to other people help you reduce stress?

Many studies have confirmed that separations from other family members, especially death and divorce, are among the most stressful events in your life. But researchers are also learning that support from those round you can have an equally powerful effect in helping combat the effects of stress.

The physical and psychological benefits of support from friends and family can be dramatic. Research studies conducted over a nine-year period in California, for example, have indicated that people who have extensive networks of social support may live longer than those who do not. Other studies have suggested that social support can reduce stress symptoms following the loss of a loved one, help speed recovery from surgery and heart attacks, and alleviate the symptoms of asthma and other disorders.

As a result of these findings, researchers now believe that social support may be crucial to understanding the wide variation in individual responses to stressful situations. One study, for example, examined 109 people living near the Three Mile Island nuclear plant in the United States at the time of the disaster there in 1979. The researchers found that those residents who received little or no support from friends and neighbours suffered the most stress-related problems, even though their levels of stress hormones were no higher than those of other residents. This suggests that, even when you are responding physically to stress, support from those round you may make you better able to cope and thus avoid the consequences of chronic stress.

Can exercise help you cope with stress?

People most often exercise for purely physical reasons, yet many who exercise report that they "feel good" after vigorous exercise. Indeed, regular exercise seems to be a powerful anti-stress activity. Exercise has been shown in a number of studies to reduce anxiety levels and feelings of helplessness, depression and hostility. At the same time, regular exercise seems to stabilize personality and to increase self-

The Effects of Stress on Performance

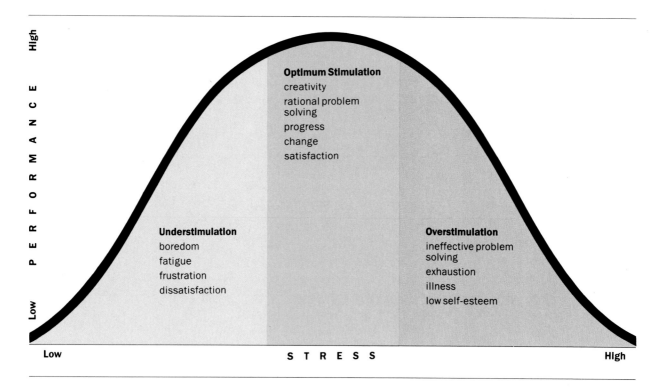

Optimum Stimulation
creativity
rational problem
solving
progress
change
satisfaction

Understimulation
boredom
fatigue
frustration
dissatisfaction

Overstimulation
ineffective problem
solving
exhaustion
illness
low self-esteem

High

P E R F O R M A N C E

Low

Low   **S T R E S S**   High

Too little stress may be as harmful as too much stress, especially if you want to get a task done. Stress researchers and students of managerial effectiveness have long recognized that some stress or stimulation is needed for optimum performance. Although the relationship between stress and performance varies from person to person, the general pattern can be expressed in the curve shown above. Performance rises as stress increases, and boredom and frustration diminish. Once an optimum point is passed, however, increasing stress impairs judgment and alertness, and performance falls off.

confidence and optimism. Exercise can even improve your sex life. According to one study, married people who embark on an exercise programme report a noticeable increase in the frequency and the quality of their sexual activity.

Even when exercise is not making you feel more relaxed, it may still be helping you to cope with stress. A recent American study compared the effect of stress on two groups of students. One group had participated in a 14-week aerobics programme; the other had not. Each group was asked to solve a set of problems and, because most of the problems were insoluble, both groups became frustrated and showed increased muscular tension and anxiety levels. However, the exercisers displayed fewer of these effects than the non-exercisers did, and they showed no increase in blood pressure, which is a key measure of stress response.

In another study (*depicted in the graph on page 21*), researchers observed the same effect. When two groups of students were subjected to a series of stressful written tests, the students who had participated in an aerobics programme had lower pulse rates than those who had not, even though both groups had reported that they felt equally stressed and anxious during the tests.

Can exercise help prevent the damage done by stress?
Exercise has also been shown to reduce many of the physical symptoms associated with stress. It has been shown, for instance, to reduce

muscle tension more effectively than some of the most commonly prescribed tranquillizers. In addition, regular vigorous exercise such as running or cycling has been shown to improve cholesterol levels in the blood and reduce the risk of hypertension and cancer. Indeed, long-term studies of nearly 17,000 Harvard University graduates have shown that those who exercise regularly have a 39 per cent lower risk of heart attack than sedentary people and that moderate exercise (the equivalent of walking 25 to 30 kilometres per week, or expending between 1,500 and 2,000 calories) can reduce the risk of death from all causes by 37 per cent.

Often, people starting out on an exercise programme to reduce stress tend to overdo it and become prematurely fatigued and perhaps injured. To best avoid injury, start out gradually at a non-competitive aerobic activity such as brisk walking, running or an aerobics routine such as the one that begins on page 70.

Do relaxation techniques alleviate stress effectively?

Yes. Simply setting time aside to learn to relax can help reduce your stress levels. A team of London researchers divided into two groups 192 men and women between the ages of 35 and 64 who had multiple risk factors for cardiovascular disease — including hypertension, high cholesterol level and a smoking habit. Both groups were given information on how to stop smoking and reduce cholesterol levels and blood pressure. In addition, one group got one hour of instruction per week on managing stress, during which it learned breathing exercises and meditation. Eight months later, the group that practised relaxation had significantly lower blood pressure and smoked fewer cigarettes than the control group. Four years later, the relaxation group had a lower incidence of hypertension and heart disease.

How will this book help you manage stress?

First, the rest of this chapter will help you assess your vulnerability to stress, summarize which stress-management techniques are effective and explain why various "quick fixes" for stress do not work. The chapters that follow will pinpoint sources of stress that you may encounter during your day — when you are getting started in the morning, during your working hours and at home during the evening. Each chapter also presents exercises and techniques that have been shown to produce positive psychological and physiological effects in coping with stress. These techniques — which include aerobics, stretching, meditation, Yoga, massage, back relaxers, progressive relaxation, imaging and biofeedback — are simple to learn and easy to incorporate into your life.

To see if you can benefit from learning some of these techniques to manage your stress better, turn to the following page.

Most people regard accidents as just that — unpredictable, isolated events. But in a study of 164 patients who had been disabled by industrial accidents, it was found that the patients scored 25 per cent higher than a normal control population on the Holmes-Rahe scale. Because the mishaps removed patients from the stresses of their jobs, it was theorized that accidents may be a misguided coping mechanism to alleviate stress.

How to Design Your Own Programme

The symptoms of stress can range from vague feelings of anxiety to lowered resistance to disease. On this page is an easy test you can take to see how much stress you may be under. This test, like the quiz on the facing page, was developed by American psychologists Lyle H. Miller and Alma Dell Smith. Clinical studies have shown that the anticipation of stress sometimes can be even more burdensome than the actual experience of it, so this test gets you to score both past and expected experiences of stress.

Check your symptoms. Give yourself a score for only those items that apply: a 1 indicates the item is not stressful; a 5 indicates that it is very stressful. Add the scores in each category, then total your scores for past and future. If your total is 30 or below, you need have little concern about the amount of stress you are under — though you may want to reduce even that. If your score is over 30, you should have some concern; and if your score is more than 53, you should be seriously concerned and think about how you can effectively manage stress.

Are You Under Stress?

PAST

If an item below affected you in the last six months, circle the number that describes the amount of stress it caused you.

1 2 3 4 5   1. Feeling that things are getting out of control

1 2 3 4 5   2. Anxiety or panic

1 2 3 4 5   3. Frustration

1 2 3 4 5   4. Anger and irritation

1 2 3 4 5   5. Feeling desperate, hopeless

1 2 3 4 5   6. Feeling trapped, helpless

1 2 3 4 5   7. Feeling depressed

1 2 3 4 5   8. Feeling guilty

1 2 3 4 5   9. Feeling self-conscious

1 2 3 4 5   10. Feeling restless

Past Score = _____

FUTURE

If you anticipate an item affecting you in the next six months, circle the number that describes the amount of stress it may cause you.

1 2 3 4 5   1. Feeling that things are getting out of control

1 2 3 4 5   2. Anxiety or panic

1 2 3 4 5   3. Frustration

1 2 3 4 5   4. Anger and irritation

1 2 3 4 5   5. Feeling desperate, hopeless

1 2 3 4 5   6. Feeling trapped, helpless

1 2 3 4 5   7. Feeling depressed

1 2 3 4 5   8. Feeling guilty

1 2 3 4 5   9. Feeling self-conscious

1 2 3 4 5   10. Feeling restless

Future Score = _____

How Stress-Resistant Are You?

1 2 3 4 5   1. I eat at least one hot, balanced meal a day.

1 2 3 4 5   2. I get seven to eight hours of sleep at least four nights a week.

1 2 3 4 5   3. I give and receive affection regularly.

1 2 3 4 5   4. I have at least one relative within 75 kilometres of home on whom I can rely.

1 2 3 4 5   5. I exercise to the point of perspiration at least twice weekly.

1 2 3 4 5   6. I limit myself to 10 cigarettes a day.

1 2 3 4 5   7. I take fewer than five alcoholic drinks a week.

1 2 3 4 5   8. I am the appropriate weight for my height and build.

1 2 3 4 5   9. My income covers my basic expenses.

1 2 3 4 5   10. I get strength from my religious beliefs.

1 2 3 4 5   11. I regularly attend social activities.

1 2 3 4 5   12. I have a network of close friends and acquaintances.

1 2 3 4 5   13. I have one or more friends to confide in about personal matters.

1 2 3 4 5   14. I am in good health (including eyesight, hearing, teeth).

1 2 3 4 5   15. I am able to speak openly about my feelings when angry or worried.

1 2 3 4 5   16. I discuss domestic problems — chores and money, for example — with the members of my household.

1 2 3 4 5   17. I have fun at least once a week.

1 2 3 4 5   18. I can organize my time effectively.

1 2 3 4 5   19. I drink fewer than three cups of coffee (or other caffeine-rich beverages) a day.

1 2 3 4 5   20. I take some quiet time for myself during the day.

Total Score = _____

No one can avoid stress altogether, but some people may be better equipped to handle stress than others; for example, those who are able to communicate openly with friends and family seem to deal well with stress. The quiz on this page will give you an idea of how resistant you are to stress, or how vulnerable.

Rate each item on the test from 1 (almost always) to 5 (never), according to how the statement pertains to you. Mark each item, even if it does not apply to you (for instance, if you do not smoke, give yourself a 1, not a 0). Add up your score.

If your total is 45 or below, you probably have excellent resistance to stress. A score over 45 indicates some vulnerability to stress, and a score over 55 indicates serious vulnerability to stress. You can strengthen your resistance to stress — and help ease the symptoms you may already have — by following the regimens in this book. To see which regimens are best suited to you, turn the page.

Colour and Stress

BLACK

The body may be less stimulated by black than by other colours. Using the level of oxygen in the blood as a measure of awareness or arousal, researchers found that people looking at a black surface had lower oxygen levels than those exposed to any other colour.

BLUE

Blue may elevate mood. In one study of university students, a higher proportion of students tested in a room lined with blue fabric described themselves as calm and happy than did those tested in rooms lined with red, yellow and neutral fabrics.

BROWN

Brown may be calming. In one study, the blood pressure levels of handicapped students were lowest during the time they spent in a classroom containing shades of brown.

GREEN

Research suggests that green may actually increase stress. In one study, people looked at coloured lights while the electrical conductivity of their skin was measured. When exposed to green light, their skin became sweatier and its electrical resistance decreased, indicating that the stress from green lights was greater than from lights of any other colour.

PINK

Studies indicate that pink may have such tranquillizing effects as lowering blood pressure, pulse rate and anxiety levels. After holding areas at a U.S. Navy prison were painted pink, researchers noted a marked decrease in prisoners' aggression and hostility.

RED

Research confirms that red is an arousing, stimulating colour. In one study, some volunteers showed dramatic changes in brain alpha waves, indicating arousal, when exposed to red light. And in a study on risk-taking conducted at a British university, students who sat under red lights gambled more and made "riskier" bets than those who sat under blue lights.

YELLOW

Yellow may reduce boredom. In one study of students listening to tapes of words repeated over and over, those students seated in areas painted yellow described themselves as more alert than those seated in areas painted in nine other colours.

How Colour Affects Stress

The colour of your surroundings can both create stress and ease the stresses in your life, often in ways that are so subtle that you are influenced subliminally (below the threshold of consciousness). Although the study of bodily responses to colour is still in its infancy, scientists in recent years have made some striking discoveries. They have shown, for example, that red light can cause seizure-like brain-wave abnormalities in epileptics and that blue light can cure jaundice in premature babies. Such findings have encouraged researchers to study the effects of colour and light on healthy individuals. Much of this research suggests that physiological responses to stress such as blood pressure, pulse and brain-wave patterns vary in an orderly manner as the colour to which people are exposed changes from red, the most stimulating colour, to blue, the least stimulating.

At the same time, many of the effects of colour on our moods may be the result of social and psychological associations with a particular colour. Red, for example, is often associated with fire and blood and is used as a colour of warning in signs. These associations vary from person to person and from culture to culture, making it difficult to choose colours that will reduce stress in everyone. But many people may be able to moderate the stimulation of a room or of clothing by the colours they choose. Where you want a stimulating effect, emphasize reds and yellows, where you want a calming influence, choose blues and browns.

Some experts believe that, as with other forms of stimulation, you may become less responsive to colours with the same effects if you allow them to predominate. So surrounding yourself with a variety of colours is probably a good idea.

Quick Fixes

The remedies that people routinely turn to when they experience stress offer relief in a variety of ways, as the chart on the right shows. Although these remedies may bring a measure of relief immediately, all of them are ultimately ineffective in reducing stress, and some may even be counterproductive and end up increasing it.

Coffee and cigarettes are among the "quick fixes" that have this conflicting effect. The caffeine in coffee and the nicotine in cigarettes both stimulate the body's neuroendocrine system. In doing so, they mimic in many ways the biochemical effects caused by physical stressors (see illustration, page 12). Among these effects are increased blood pressure and pulse rate, and the secretion of hormones such as adrenaline, which prepares the body for fight or flight. Because caffeine and nicotine produce feelings of alertness and energy, and sometimes even euphoria, you may want to reach for a cigarette or a cup of coffee when you are under stress. However, these same chemicals can also increase tension and anxiety, and thereby boost your level of stress.

Alcoholic drinks, tranquillizers and sleeping pills have a very different effect. They depress many of the same bodily functions that coffee and cigarettes stimulate. For this reason, they can ease the anxiety and tension that are often associated with stressful events. But they also slow reaction time and impair coordination and judgment. And their prolonged use can lead to chronic depression and still more anxiety.

Perhaps the most stressful of the effects of these quick fixes is their tendency to cause habituation or even addiction when used for prolonged periods. Some researchers believe that this may be partly the result of their effects on the biochemistry of stress. Both nicotine and alcohol, for example, have been shown to enhance the effect of endorphins, the body's natural opiates, relieving pain and anxiety and causing feelings of pleasure. Some researchers believe that people continue to use quick fixes, eventually becoming dependent on them, to prolong these pleasurable effects and to avoid the unpleasant sensations that may occur when use of these substances is stopped.

Most of the remedies shown in the chart, except coffee, are also used to help cope with another of the most common symptoms of stress: difficulty falling asleep or the lack of restful sleep. Alcohol and the various tranquillizers, especially the barbiturates, are often effective in bringing on sleep. However, even short-term use disturbs sleep patterns, often causing light sleep with frequent awakenings. For advice on how to get a good night's sleep, see pages 118-119.

Dietary quick fixes for stress, represented here by milk, herbal teas, chocolate and stress vitamins, are certainly safer than stimulants or sedatives. The most heavily promoted nutritional remedy for stress, so-called stress vitamins, has been shown by many studies to have no effect on stress except in cases of injury or other *physical* stress. The best dietary remedy for handling stress is a balanced diet that follows the guidelines presented in Chapter Five of this book.

How Not to Manage Stress

QUICK FIX	LASTING EFFECTS
For normal social drinkers (two drinks a day or less), **alcohol** induces relaxation and mild elation; for heavy drinkers it can produce anxiety, depression and disturbed sleep patterns.	For normal social drinkers, gradual tolerance diminishes feelings of relaxation and elation; continued use by heavy drinkers can lead to heart disease, liver disease, brain dysfunction, cancer and permanently disordered sleep.
The sugar content of **chocolate** produces a temporary rise in blood sugar, resulting in feelings of energy followed by an insulin "backlash" that causes lassitude, irritability and fatigue. (Chocolate also contains caffeine — see coffee.)	Sugar content may contribute to dental cavities, cause weight gain and help induce diabetes in susceptible people.
The caffeine in **coffee** improves alertness and reaction time, and may enhance concentration and dexterity; more than three cups a day can stimulate secretion of stomach acid and cause digestive upset; late-night consumption can delay or disrupt sleep.	Gradual tolerance develops, which diminishes stimulating effects; more than three cups a day may lead to irregular heartbeat, headaches, muscle tension, irritability and insomnia.
In moderate amounts as a substitute for coffee or caffeine-containing teas, **herbal teas** can be pleasant and can soothe digestion (unless you have an allergy to a particular herb).	Many herbs are powerful drugs that can cause unpredictable reactions and should not be consumed without medical advice.
A traditional remedy for insomnia, warm **milk** contains the amino acid L-tryptophan, which the body uses to produce sleep-regulating chemicals; few researchers now believe, however, that taking extra L-tryptophan in any form can help induce sleep.	It has no lasting stress-related effects.
Sleeping pills produce a feeling of relaxation and act on the brain to induce a sleep whose patterns closely resemble those of natural sleep.	They can disturb the pattern of sleep in the same manner as tranquillizers but less severely; they can cause lethargy and impaired performance during waking periods.
The so-called **stress vitamins** — vitamin C and the B vitamins — may be necessary during *physical* stress (during pregnancy, after surgery or during certain drug therapies, for example), but they are useless for short-term mental or psychological stress.	When the body responds to physical stress by suppressing the appetite, a healthy, balanced diet — or, in extreme cases, a vitamin-mineral supplement — can prevent harmful nutrient depletion; replacing only vitamin C and the B vitamins will do no good.
The nicotine in **tobacco** stimulates the production of adrenaline and other hormones, increasing alertness, relieving anxiety and producing a feeling of energy; tobacco smoke can stain teeth and cause breathlessness and dizziness.	Prolonged use of tobacco impairs circulation and respiration and disturbs sleep patterns; it also increases the risk of a variety of cancers, as well as the risk of cardiac disease.
Tranquillizers relieve anxiety, produce a feeling of relaxation and can help induce sleep; they also slow respiration and nervous-system function, and are extremely dangerous in large doses or in combination with alcohol and other drugs.	When taken for more than three days, they can cause lethargy during waking periods, aggravate insomnia, decrease periods of deep sleep and even cause nightmares; protracted use can lead to drug dependence, fatigue and feelings of depression.

Stress-Reducing Exercises

AEROBICS
pages 70-77

This is associated with a lower resting heart rate and reduced risk of hypertension, muscle tenseness, depression, anxiety, obesity and stroke; a midday aerobics programme is a powerful stress reliever.

BACK RELAXERS
pages 92-95

Stretching and strengthening exercises can alleviate lower back pain produced by muscular tension, stress and poor posture; a few minutes of exercise can relieve symptoms in 80 per cent of all back-pain cases.

BIOFEEDBACK
pages 80-81

Blood pressure, muscle tension and skin temperature can be lowered when the subject concentrates on relaxing; this may reduce hypertension, relieve headache and diminish other symptoms of stress and anxiety.

IMAGING
pages 78-79

This technique is similar to one that athletes use to improve their performance; individuals imagine themselves in pleasant or relaxing situations to improve their sense of relaxation; this is also an effective treatment for hypertension.

JAW RELAXERS
pages 102-103

These can reduce or eliminate bruxism, an unconscious grinding and clenching of the teeth that is a symptom of stress and results in facial pain, toothache, periodontal disease, displacement of the teeth, locking of the jaw and muscle spasms.

LOW-STRESS POSTURE
pages 60-61

Poor posture can result in mechanical imbalances that lead to muscular tension, headache, dizziness and joint damage; improving sitting and standing postures can increase respiratory capacity and lessen the chance of developing spinal deformities.

MASSAGE
pages 48-51, 68-69, 90-91, 96-101

This can effectively reduce such symptoms of stress as muscular tension, hypertension and anxiety; it can also promote sound sleep in people who suffer from chronic stress-related sleeping disorders.

MEDITATION
pages 52-53

This powerful relaxer has been shown to reduce symptoms of bronchial asthma, hypertension and anxiety; it may also relieve chronic pain as well as headache.

PROGRESSIVE RELAXATION
pages 116-117

This involves tensing and relaxing major muscle groups from the face to the toes; it has been shown to lower high blood pressure and reduce feelings of tension and anxiety.

SLEEP POSITIONS
pages 118-119

These take pressure off the spine and promote relaxation; special support is needed for reading or watching television in bed because inadequate neck and back support often induces tension and makes it more difficult to fall asleep.

STRETCHING
pages 38-41, 58-59, 62-67, 76-77, 92-95

This can reduce muscular tension, improve posture and increase a sense of relaxation; it helps prevent or relieve muscular pain that results from overusing muscles.

TAI CHI
pages 42-47

This consists of dancelike movements designed to promote good physical and mental health; it instils a feeling of calmness; it is an exercise for every part of the body.

WATER RELAXATION
pages 82-83

This involves either suspension in a flotation tank or floating in a warm, calm salt-water pool; it can decrease the presence of stress hormones in the blood, lower blood pressure and ease muscle tension.

YOGA
pages 104-115

Practitioners are able to decrease heart rate, respiration and certain brain-wave activities to achieve deep relaxation without inducing drowsiness or sleep.

Choosing an Exercise

Experts in the field of stress management increasingly regard exercise as the safest and healthiest way to reduce stress. The exercises in this book, shown opposite, include both general routines to reduce stress levels and more specific exercises that target certain symptoms. Although studies show that many types of exercise — stretching, meditation, aerobics and massage — reduce stress, not every exercise will appeal to everyone, nor will all exercises be appropriate for every time and place. Studies show that those who experience stress-related illness or symptoms of stress can best reduce or eliminate those symptoms with a programme of stress management that includes exercise. Since you are more likely to stick with an exercise you enjoy than one that you find tedious, you should have a variety to choose from.

Each portion of the day confronts you with its own set of stressors. And certain exercises are best suited for specific times of the day. Therefore, the exercises of this book are distributed among morning, daytime and evening chapters. This does not mean that you are limited to performing, say, the lunch-time aerobics workout on pages 70-77 during your lunch hour or even during the daytime. But you may find that your lunch hour is a convenient time to do this workout. Similarly, you do not have to wait until evening to perform the progressive-relaxation exercises which are described on pages 116-117. But because they are designed to be performed lying down, you will probably find that it is most convenient to do them near bedtime and that they provide an excellent way for you to unwind at the end of the day.

CHAPTER TWO

Getting Started

Circadian rhythms — a key to morning stress

One of the major factors that determine how you start the day — feeling relaxed, cheerful and alert, or sluggish, irritable and unable to concentrate — is a set of biological fluctuations called circadian rhythms (from the Latin words *circa* and *dies*, meaning "about the day"). These include daily cycles of sleep and wakefulness, hunger, cardiovascular activity, hormone levels and body temperature. Circadian rhythms are regulated by a complex network of biochemical clocks, and a number of the rhythms are synchronized: your body temperature, for example, normally drops as you sleep, then rises — albeit by as little as half a degree Celsius during the day. As it rises, your mood becomes elevated, and your alertness and ability to perform rise as well.

If you could live each day in accordance with your circadian rhythms, you would wake up feeling refreshed, energetic and ready to cope with stressful events, both anticipated and unanticipated. Unfortunately, this degree of harmony is difficult to achieve, partly because many circadian rhythms do not follow the earth's 24-hour cycle of day and night. This was discovered when researchers placed people underground for long periods under constant lighting and found that the subjects' temperature and other bodily functions followed a 25-hour cycle. The result was that the subjects began falling asleep and waking up an hour later each day. Under normal conditions, however, such cues as morning sunlight, mealtimes and the activities of other people reset your circadian clocks daily to a 24-hour cycle, a process scientists call entrainment.

Although your body can adapt to a 24-hour cycle, it cannot cope with major or abrupt changes in sleeping and waking patterns without signs of stress. Research has shown that human beings can comfortably shift their circadian cycle by no more than one or two hours a day; furthermore, it is easier to shift forwards (probably because of our 25-hour cycle) than backwards, so that your body prefers going to bed a little later each day and rising a little later. One example of circadian disruption has been studied extensively — the common air traveller's complaint of jet lag. If the change in time zones is more than a few hours, your circadian cycle may have to drift all the way round the clock to get back in phase, a process that may take at least a week. While this adjustment is taking place, you will probably experience fatigue, weakness, headache and irritability, along with reductions in cognitive and psychomotor performance.

Dramatic effects of this kind have also been shown in workers who rotate working hours daily or weekly, especially when they must move to an earlier shift. When the schedules of 85 workers at an American factory were altered so that their shifts rotated less frequently and moved forwards rather than backwards, staff turnover decreased and productivity rose by 22 per cent. The near-catastrophic accident at the Three Mile Island nuclear power plant in 1979 occurred at 4 a.m. on a day following an employee shift rotation — and poor performance has been implicated as a major contributory factor in that accident.

You cannot ignore the effects of your body's circadian rhythms. But you can take steps which will help to synchronize these cycles more smoothly — primarily by establishing regular habits — and make the cycles conform more closely to the demands of your day with little or no distress, so that your body is willing to wake up and perform when you need it to.

Studies have shown that irregular waking and sleeping patterns will upset your circadian rhythms more than missing sleep will. If you have missed some sleep, therefore, it is better not to try to make it up with extra sleep the next night. Keeping a regular waking-up schedule seven days a week is the best way to establish a consistent circadian pattern. To ease the transition between sleep and waking, try the gentle stretches on pages 38-41. A mildly stimulating self-massage such as the Do-in (pronounced doe-EEN) on pages 48-51 can help dissipate early-morning grogginess.

Exercise and Body Temperature

Your body temperature fluctuates according to your physical activities and circadian rhythms, starting at around 36°C early in the morning. Since mental alertness and physical performance are often linked to circadian rhythms and body temperature, people who engage in such vigorous exercises as running or cycling in the morning may find that these activities can overcome early-morning lows of temperature and alertness.

When you exercise, your body temperature may rise to around 38°C. After you stop, your temperature gradually returns to normal. Exercise will not change the timetable of your circadian rhythms, but it will overcome the rhythms for a time. The chart on the right represents how this works.

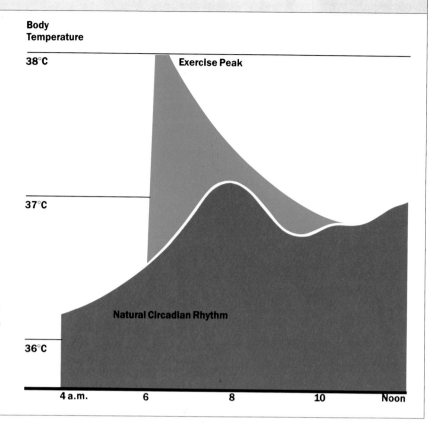

Body Temperature

38°C — Exercise Peak

37°C

Natural Circadian Rhythm

36°C

4 a.m.   6   8   10   Noon

Meditation *(pages 52-53)* is another way to start the day calmly. By shifting the mind away from logical, externally orientated thoughts, meditation can produce a systemic effect on the minds and bodies of those who practise it: studies show that it markedly reduces heart, respiration and metabolic rates while affecting brain-wave patterns. Tai Chi (pronounced tie-GEE), shown in a routine on pages 42-47, has been practised in the Orient for centuries as an exercise, a dance, a relaxation technique and a religious ritual. Tai Chi warms up your muscles without stress. It can even be done as a gentle aerobic exercise if it is sustained for 30 minutes — and some evidence shows that morning is the optimum time for an aerobic workout *(see chart above)*.

Finally, although the evidence is inconclusive that skipping breakfast causes stress or impairs performance, there are some reasons to play it safe and start the day with a good meal. In the morning, your body is switching from a stage of low energy expenditure, lower temperature and low hormone production into its more active daytime mode, and it seems prudent to support this change-over with the right nutrients. The timing of your breakfast is not important — it can be eaten first thing in the morning or, if you prefer, later on. But eating breakfast at the same time every day will keep your circadian rhythms functioning smoothly, which in turn lets you manage stress better throughout the day.

Waking-Up
Stretches/1

When you wake up in the morning, many of the functions controlled by your body's circadian rhythms have only just started to accelerate. Your heart rate is still slow, your body temperature is relatively low, your muscles are stiff and your mind is not yet fully alert. Rather than reaching for a stimulant like coffee or dashing to catch a bus, take five minutes to perform a series of morning stretches. These stretches will not only gently rouse your neuro-muscular system, but they will help you maintain a sense of relaxation.

Never jerk your muscles or force a stretch. Ease into a stretch slowly until you feel a pleasant elongation of the muscles. Then extend the stretch a little farther. You can lengthen a muscle to the point of mild discomfort, but you should never feel pain when you stretch. Hold the stretch for 10 to 30 seconds and relax. Repeat the exercise two or three times for maximum effectiveness. If a stretch shown in this chapter involves only one limb or one side of the body, perform the same stretch with the other limb or on the opposite side as well.

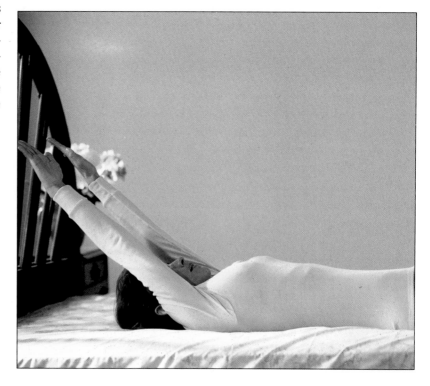

When you wake up in the morning, lie on your back and extend your hands towards the ceiling *(right, top).* **Then slowly swing your hands in an arc above your head** *(right, bottom)* **until they lie flat on the mattress, stretching both your chest and shoulder muscles.**

Remain on your back and grasp your right knee, drawing it towards your chest *(above)*. This will stretch your buttocks and your hamstrings, a group of muscles along the back of the thigh. Pull both knees to your chest *(below)* to stretch the lower back.

As you are getting out of bed, perform these four stretches. To stretch the muscles along your entire back, kneel on the bed and place your buttocks on your heels *(below)*. Rest your forehead on the mattress and place your hands at your sides, palms turned up. Next, sit on the bed with your left hand on the mattress and your right hand pressed against your left knee *(right, top)*. Turn your body to the left to stretch the muscles on your right side, then repeat for the left side. Get off the bed, grasp the underside of the bed frame and squat down to stretch the hamstrings, buttocks and lower back *(right, centre)*. Finally, lie on the floor with a towel or pillow under your pelvis for comfort *(right, bottom)*. With your hands and forearms resting on the floor, raise your elbows about five centimetres. Looking directly ahead, lift your head gently to stretch your chest and abdominal muscles.

A Set of Tai Chi

Mastering Tai Chi requires a knowledgeable teacher. But you can get a good sense of Tai Chi's benefits by moving through this sequence of 45 classic postures, shown with their Chinese names on these two pages and the following four. Practise three or four movements at a time until you can perform them fluidly. Then move on to another short sequence. Note the positions of hands and feet, and keep your back straight. For comfort, wear loose-fitting clothing and slippers or aerobics shoes.

Start out standing erect. Turn your right foot out 45 degrees and sink down slightly on your right leg. Shift all your weight on to that leg and extend your left leg, flexing your foot and crossing your hands in front of your chest (1). Step back on to your left foot, turning it out, and move your hands to waist level as you shift your weight to the left leg (2). Swing your arms to the right and press forwards, shifting some of your weight to the right leg (3). Pivot left, shifting your weight to your right leg, bringing your left foot round and opening your arms (4). Step forwards, leading with your right leg (5). Your right hand, elbow, knee and toes should be in alignment. Slide your left foot forwards and move your right arm parallel to the floor (6). Step back on your left foot as you raise your left hand and twist to the right (7). Step back on your right foot (8); parry with your left arm and punch with your right. Rock back on to your right leg and bring your arms up (9). Pivot 90 degrees to the right, crossing your arms (10). Slide forwards, dropping your left hand to waist level and extending your right hand (11). Step back with your left foot and straighten your right leg and arm (12). Pivot and step out, opening your arms (13). Come forwards, shifting your weight to your right leg, and extend your left arm (14). Then pivot and step out with your left foot, moving your right hand up to your temple (15).

1. Salutation to the Buddha

2. Grasp Bird's Tail

6. White Crane Spreads Its Wings

7. Brush, Knee, Twist, Step

11. Fist under Elbow

12. Repulse Monkey

Grasp Bird's Tail

4. Single Whip

5. White Crane Spreads Its Wings

. Parry, Punch

9. Closing

10. Embracing Tiger

13. Diagonal Flying

14. Raise Left Hand

15. Fan through the Arms

Tai Chi/2

Pivot right (16). Step up, with knees bent, and push out with hands flexed (17). Pivot right, so that you face straight ahead, and extend your left leg out as your arms and torso rotate right (18). Rotate to the left as you bring your feet together (19). Rotate right and then left four times, ending in a single whip position (*see position 4*). Rotate your torso right and kick your right leg straight out as you open your arms (20). Shift your weight to your right leg and kick with your left (21). Lower your leg almost to the floor, turn your right foot out and kick again with your left leg (22). Drop your left leg back, shift your weight on to it and parry high and low with your arms (23). Pivot on your left foot and switch hand positions (24). Then pivot on your right foot, jump on to your left foot and kick your right leg — taking care to avoid straining — towards your extended right arm (25). Step back on your right leg, drop your arms and shift backwards on to your left foot (26). Pivot in a full circle, coming round to stand on your left leg, and kick with your right (27). Drop down, bending your left leg and keeping your right leg straight and your feet parallel; cover your right wrist with your left palm (28). Swing your right leg back and open your arms (29). Step forwards, moving your fists to your chest and hip (30).

16. Green Dragon Dropping Water

17. Step Up and Push

21. Separation of Legs

22. Separation of Legs

26. Step Back, Hands to the Side

27. Kick with the Sole

18. Cloud Hands

19. Cloud Hands

20. Separation of Legs

23. Wind Blowing Lotus

24. Wind Blowing Lotus

25. Double Jump Kick

28. Clap Opponent with Fist

29. Diagonal Single Whip

30. Parting of Wild Horse's Mane

Tai Chi/3

Begin the Fair Lady Works the Shuttles (31 and 32) by turning to one side. Parry with one hand and punch with the other. Then pivot 90 degrees to your left and punch and parry again. Repeat the 90-degree pivot, along with the punch and parry, two more times, bringing you full circle. Finish with a single whip (*see position 4*). Shift your weight to your right leg and extend your torso and left arm towards your left foot (33). Swing round to face left; shift your weight on to your left leg and raise your right leg (34). Extend your right leg straight out and step forwards. Turn and block your temple with your left hand as you move your right arm and leg forwards (35). Step on to your right foot. Bring your arms out in loose fists, as though you were boxing an opponent's ears (36). Then repeat the stepping movement and punch both fists in an uppercut (37). Step on to your left foot and kick your right leg high and slightly left, so that it moves across your extended palms (38). Step to bring your feet into a T position (39), drop your right fist directly down and block up with your left hand. Pivot to face left, sink down on your left leg and punch and parry at chest level (40). Extend your right leg and arm back in a reverse lunge (41). Shift back on to your right leg and pivot to face forwards, extending your right arm (42). Follow up with two short punches (43). Form a mirror image of position 2, but with your forward foot flexed (44). Swing your hands up, crossing your palms at chest level, then lower your arms and turn so that you face forwards (45).

31. Fair Lady Works the Shuttles

32. Fair Lady Works the Shuttles

36. Cannon through the Sky

37. Cannon through the Sky

41. Retreat to Ride the Tiger

42. Turn the Moon

3. Single Whip Down

34. Golden Cock Stands on One Leg

35. Cannon through the Sky

38. Lotus Kick

39. Downward Punch

40. Step Up to Form Seven Stars

43. Shoot Tiger with Bow

44. Grasp Bird's Tail

45. Conclusion

Morning Massage/1

Derived from an Oriental rejuvenation and healing technique called Do-in, the stimulating yet gentle massage here and on pages 50-51 involves lightly rapping or drumming yourself with your knuckles. This technique helps stimulate blood flow to the muscles, the connective tissues such as tendons and ligaments, and the tissues near your skin. You can use the technique virtually anywhere on your body that you can reach.

It is not necessary to hit yourself forcefully. Make a loose fist and keep your wrist flexible, then swing your hand back and forth to produce a light drumming motion.

Keep your wrists flexible and rhythmically tap your knuckles on the top and sides of your head, moving over your entire scalp.

As a warm-up, grab a handful of hair with each hand and tug for five seconds. Then grab two more handfuls and continue the process until you have stimulated your entire scalp.

Drum lightly down the back of your neck and progress along your right shoulder with the left hand. Repeat on the left side.

Continue drumming over the top of your left shoulder and progress along your upper arm to the elbow. Repeat on the right side.

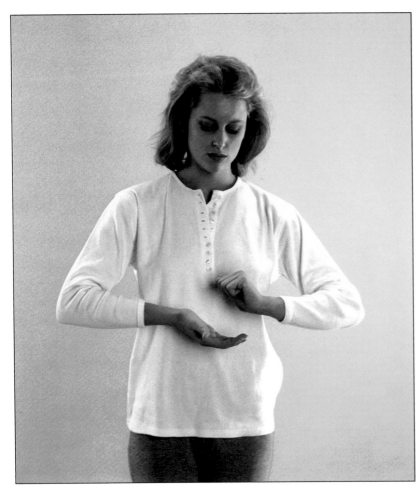

Gently strike your forearm, moving down its entire length. Open your hand and continue rapping on your palm and fingers.

Kneel on the floor and sit on your heels. Rap with both fists on the inside of your left thigh. Repeat on the right thigh.

Gently drum up and down the ribs along your back. Stay close to your spine without actually striking it.

Complete your self-massage with this relaxing deep-breathing exercise. Sit on your heels and bring your hands together *(left)*. Exhale forcefully, then inhale slowly as you draw your right arm out to the side; pretend there is tension on your arm as though you were stretching a large rubber band. When your arm is fully extended your lungs should be full of air. Open your hand and release the band as you exhale and release tension *(above)*. Repeat for your left arm.

Remain kneeling but rise up off your heels *(opposite)*. Strike your buttocks with both fists. Because your muscles and flesh are thicker here than elsewhere, you can drum more forcefully.

Morning Meditation

There are many philosophies of meditation, each with its own set of techniques. But Dr. Herbert Benson of the Harvard Medical School, who has studied meditation as a means of reducing stress, has outlined four steps that can trigger the relaxation response (*see page 18*) as effectively as techniques used by experienced meditators. Dr. Benson recommends meditating for 10 to 20 minutes in the morning and again later in the day. Each time, you should follow these simple guidelines.

First, you need a quiet environment where you will not be distracted or disturbed. Some people find that darkening a room or closing their eyes helps them meditate, while others prefer a dimly lit space. And some meditators want silence, while others prefer a background of soft music or sounds.

Second, a comfortable position is important — one that you can assume for at least 20 minutes without feeling strained or numb and one that also keeps you from falling asleep. Each position shown here is well suited for this.

Third, you need a device to fix your attention on. This can be a mantra — a word, sound or phrase repeated each time you exhale. Or you can fix your gaze on a stationary object. Breathing slowly and rhythmically will also help you to focus your thoughts.

Finally, adopt a passive attitude: do not worry about how well you are doing. At first your mind may wander, but with some practice you will be able to focus for longer periods, enhancing your ability to produce the response.

To meditate in a lotus position, sit cross-legged on the floor and place each foot on the opposite thigh. Place your hands on your knees with palms facing up. This position keeps the spine erect and the chest open for relaxed breathing.

If the lotus is too difficult for you to perform, you may still be able to meditate comfortably seated cross-legged. Keep your body upright and your arms relaxed. Your hands should not grasp your knees but rest gently on them.

Meditate in a sitting position either in a chair *(above)* or on a meditating stool *(below)*. The chair should allow you to sit comfortably erect with your feet flat on the floor; the stool should be slanted so that you can keep your back and head straight when you kneel.

CHAPTER THREE

Nine to Five

Strategies for coping with the emotional and physical pressures at work

W hether its source is a tyranni-
cal boss, a harried journey to the office or a pressing deadline, stress is
all too often a part of the working day. Unlike morning stress, which
tends to be generated internally, much job-related stress comes from
external forces that are difficult, if not impossible, to control.

A major study of 657 blue and white-collar workers at a large car
factory identified four factors that can lead to stress in the workplace:
overload, which may include a heavy volume of work and restrictive
rules; low job satisfaction; little influence over one's work situation;
and conflicts with co-workers and supervisors. Other investigations
yield similar findings: jobs that tangle you up in red tape, wear you
down with meaningless chores or require you to handle complaints
from clients and customers lead to stress and stress-related illnesses.
The U.S. Federal Aviation Administration's psychology laboratory
found that fast-paced air-traffic control — what many people would
consider an extremely demanding situation — was actually the least
stressful, most rewarding aspect of the controllers' jobs; shifting
schedules and irrelevant work created the most stress. An American survey of police officers revealed that dramatic car chases

and confrontations with criminals — even shootouts — ranked far behind excessive paperwork and an "ineffectual judicial system" as sources of job stress.

Poor motivation, fatigue and drug use can sometimes be traced to monotonous and impersonal jobs. A study of sawmill workers in boring, assembly-line jobs revealed that they had much more adrenaline in their blood than did sawmill employees who did not work on the assembly line. Furthermore, the adrenaline level of the bored employees increased during the course of the working day, an indication of rising stress. And those least satisfied with their jobs had difficulty relaxing after work and tended to have the highest absenteeism, with problems ranging from chest pains to depression.

Whatever stresses are present in the workplace, a good boss can minimize their effects. This was dramatically illustrated by a study of working conditions at an American telephone company: employees who were under stress but who had supportive bosses reported half as many illnesses as those who said their families — not their bosses — gave them their support. Furthermore, those who received little support from their bosses were ill more often than those who said they received little support from their families. According to experts, a good boss can help his or her employees cope with stress, not by solving their problems for them but by giving them the tools with which to solve them on their own.

Not all of these nine-to-five stresses are caused by the emotional factors of a job. Indeed, a person may be perfectly happy at his job and still suffer from stresses caused by environmental conditions, such as poor lighting and ventilation, excessive noise and inadequate or excessive heating. Even such simple factors as poorly adjusted chairs and glare from a video display terminal can cause stress. A U.S. government survey of clerks who worked intensively at video display terminals found that these workers suffered higher-than-average eye strain, as well as high levels of stress.

One of the best ways to reduce emotional and physical stress on the job is through regular exercise. Not only does physical activity reduce such symptoms of stress as fatigue and anxiety, but studies show that the aerobically fit are better able to cope with the chronic stresses of the workplace. In addition, those who exercise regularly have been shown to rate higher in overall job performance and productivity than those who do not. As an added benefit, exercise also improves general fitness by lowering blood pressure, reducing resting heart rate and contributing to weight loss.

Some companies have experimented with exercise programmes as a way to increase productivity and to reduce sick leave and corporate health-care expenditures. The results of one such study showed that adherence to an exercise programme boosted worker productivity and reduced absenteeism. In another study, an insurance company conducted a five-year survey of 1,389 office workers, most of whom had

Avoiding Afternoon Slump

◆ Workers frequently complain of low energy and loss of concentration late in the afternoon. Are these simply signs of fatigue? Researchers now suspect that your midday meal can contribute to an afternoon slump.

◆ A study at the University of Sussex revealed that students who ate a larger-than-average lunch (more than 1,000 calories) experienced decreased alertness and slowed reflexes, which mimicked the effects of missing a night's sleep. Why this occurred is unclear, but the process of digestion has been implicated. Apparently, the larger the meal, the more blood is diverted to the stomach for digestion, so the less there is for the rest of the body. The solution to this problem is to avoid large lunches. If you are hungry by midmorning, a light snack will take the edge off your appetite.

◆ In addition, several studies have indicated a cause-and-effect relationship between the balance of nutrients in your meal and slowdown afterwards. In one study, researchers found that eating carbohydrate-rich, protein-poor foods triggers the release of serotonin, a chemical neurotransmitter located in the brain that is associated with the onset of sleep. So, if you eat pasta for lunch, have a small amount of chicken, meat, beans or other protein as well.

◆ Keeping your food intake fairly constant from day to day may also help. People who shift back and forth from heavy to light lunches, or who skip breakfast and eat heartily at midday, are more likely to feel sluggish in mid-afternoon than those who eat moderately at regular intervals.

sedentary jobs. Those employees who engaged in a corporate physical-fitness programme showed a 46 per cent reduction in major medical costs annually, and a 36 per cent reduction in disability days (not counting maternity leave). After five years, the company realized a savings of £1.93 for each pound invested in the fitness programme. Not all companies offer comprehensive fitness programmes, of course; however, even short stretching routines to loosen up after long periods of sitting can relieve stress, according to several studies.

This chapter describes routines designed to help you cope with stress at work or on your way to work. You can take a few moments to relax during your journey to or from the office, even on a crowded bus or train or in your car, by performing the six-step stretching routine shown on pages 58-59. And the aerobics routine on pages 70-77 is a complete workout you can perform during your lunch hour.

You can also concentrate on problems of stress that are specific to your own work. If you type extensively, for instance, you will benefit from performing hand-strengthening and stretching exercises (*pages 68-69*). If, however, you spend a great deal of time either standing or sitting in one position, achieving the correct posture may reduce your stress level (*pages 60-61*). Specialized techniques such as mental imaging and biofeedback (*pages 78-81*) can also help to relieve on-the-job stress and improve job performance.

Getting to Work

A commuter deals with a multitude of stressors. Studies on animals show that even a slight environmental change is enough to alter hormone levels in the blood and to increase other chemical signs of stress. In addition to the stress of simply moving from one place to another, travel presents environmental stress in the form of car exhaust, vibration and noise, such physical stresses as the discomfort of sitting or standing in a cramped space, and the psychological stresses of uncontrollable delays such as traffic jams.

Driving is particularly stressful for many people because it exposes them to most, if not all, of the above stresses, with the additional burden of having to concentrate, particularly when driving at high speeds, in heavy traffic or in bad weather. Driving can result in a faster heart rate, increased hormone production, elevated blood pressure, sweating, nervous and muscular tension, gastrointestinal disturbances and other physiological signs of stress.

One of the easiest ways to reduce the stresses of commuting is simply to leave plenty of time to reach your destination. For a journey to the office that usually takes between 30 and 60 minutes, give yourself an extra 20 minutes or so to allow for any unexpected delays.

You can also reduce the stresses of commuting with stretching routines. Stretching can relieve tension in your neck, shoulder and back muscles, which can easily become cramped when you remain in the same position for an extended period. Perform the exercises shown here while you are seated in a bus, train or plane, or while you are stopped at a traffic light or in a traffic jam in your car. Hold each stretch for 20 seconds.

Keeping your shoulders steady, drop your head to the right, bringing your ear towards your shoulder *(above)*. Repeat, dropping your head to the left.

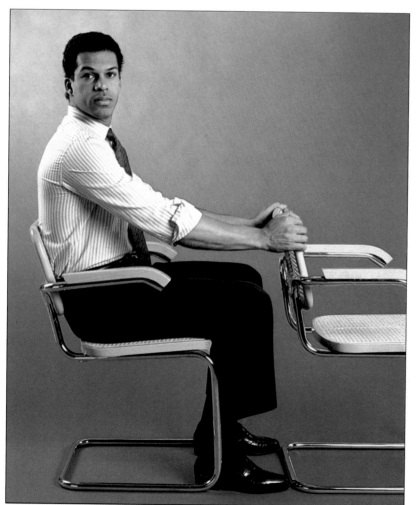

Grip the steering wheel or the seat in front of you to steady your shoulders. Turn your head to the right, stretching your neck muscles. Then turn to the left.

Bring your right hand up and draw it across your body to stretch your right shoulder. Repeat for the left shoulder.

Raise your right hand over your head and draw your right arm and shoulder back into a stretch. Repeat on the left side.

Intertwine your fingers behind your neck and bring your elbows as far back as possible. Keep your neck straight.

Place your hands against the dashboard or the back of the seat in front of you. Extend your arms and push your back into the seat.

Low-Stress Posture

Good posture conveys the impression that you are alert and confident; it can also relieve many physical stresses. Poor posture, such as slumping, hunching your shoulders and drooping your head, can lead to many health problems, including backache, sunken chest, pain in the arms, shoulders and neck, knee injury, joint strain and cartilage damage.

Ill-fitting clothing and improperly sized furniture often contribute to poor posture. Make sure that your clothing does not restrict your normal movement in any way and that your chair allows you to sit straight up comfortably. Then follow the basic guidelines given here for the correct way of holding yourself while sitting or standing.

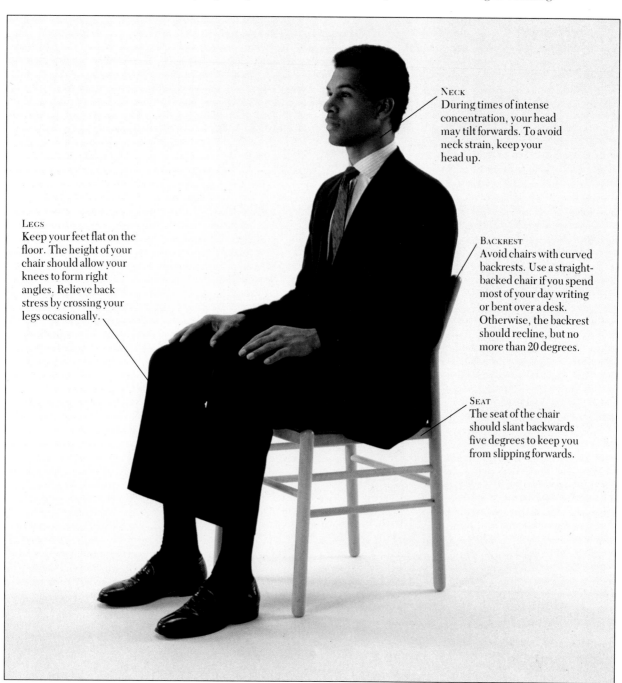

NECK
During times of intense concentration, your head may tilt forwards. To avoid neck strain, keep your head up.

LEGS
Keep your feet flat on the floor. The height of your chair should allow your knees to form right angles. Relieve back stress by crossing your legs occasionally.

BACKREST
Avoid chairs with curved backrests. Use a straight-backed chair if you spend most of your day writing or bent over a desk. Otherwise, the backrest should recline, but no more than 20 degrees.

SEAT
The seat of the chair should slant backwards five degrees to keep you from slipping forwards.

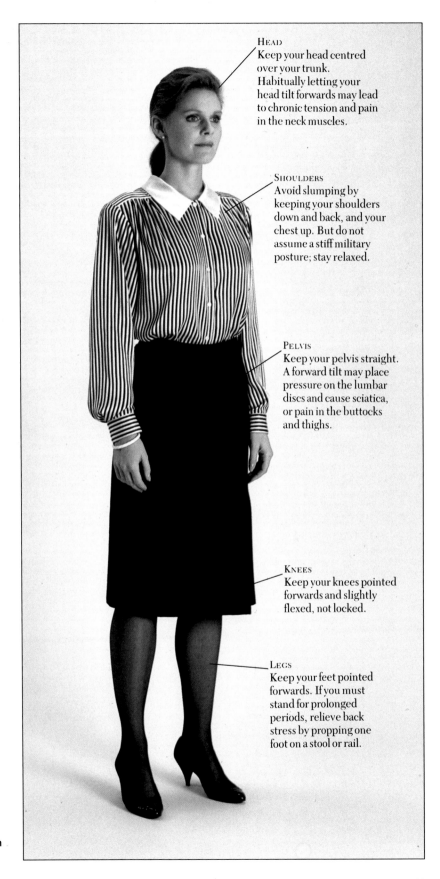

HEAD
Keep your head centred over your trunk. Habitually letting your head tilt forwards may lead to chronic tension and pain in the neck muscles.

SHOULDERS
Avoid slumping by keeping your shoulders down and back, and your chest up. But do not assume a stiff military posture; stay relaxed.

PELVIS
Keep your pelvis straight. A forward tilt may place pressure on the lumbar discs and cause sciatica, or pain in the buttocks and thighs.

KNEES
Keep your knees pointed forwards and slightly flexed, not locked.

LEGS
Keep your feet pointed forwards. If you must stand for prolonged periods, relieve back stress by propping one foot on a stool or rail.

Generally, whether you are standing or sitting, your back should be erect but not ramrod-straight. When viewed from the rear, your spine should look straight; from the side, it should form a slight S curve.

Deskbound Stretching/1

Some of the most stressful jobs involve sitting at a desk all day. In a study by the U.S. National Institute for Occupational Safety and Health, secretaries, managers and administrators were among those who suffered the highest rate of such stress-related illnesses as hypertension and heart attack. But being deskbound need not prevent you from taking a few minutes out of even the busiest day to reduce tension. In less than 15 minutes, you can perform the comprehensive relaxation routine on this page and the following five pages. These exercises will serve to reduce stress by focusing your mind on something other than anxiety-provoking job pressures. Simple distraction, studies show, can significantly reduce your level of anxiety. Of equal importance, this stretching routine will work to relieve the physical symptoms of stress, such as rapid, shallow breathing and muscular tension.

Do not bounce or jerk as you perform these stretches; do them slowly and deliberately. Be sure to breathe deeply and evenly, but never force your breath. For best results, hold each stretch for 10 to 20 seconds, relax and then repeat once or twice.

Relieve tension in your fingers and hands by extending your arms in front of you and spreading your fingers *(above)*. Then, one by one, touch the tip of each finger to your thumb *(below)*.

Interlace your fingers and grasp the back of your head. Drop your chin towards your chest and push down with your hands until you feel a stretch in the muscles along the back of your neck.

Sit fully erect in your chair and interlace your fingers behind your back. Gradually pull your arms backwards and upwards. You will stretch your chest, shoulders and upper arms.

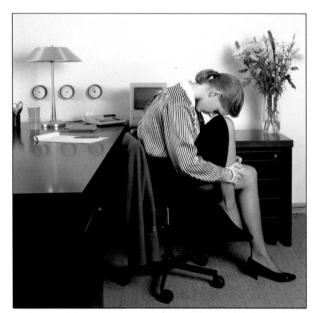

Turn your chair away from your desk and lift your right knee. Grasp your shin with your hands and pull your knee higher, touching your forehead to your knee. Repeat for the left leg.

Keep both feet flat on the floor and drop your head towards your knees. Let your arms dangle freely. This pose will relieve tension in your lower back and increase circulation to your head.

Deskbound Stretching/2

Place your arms in front of you with one hand over the other *(right)*. Turn your head to the right and pull your right elbow back so that it is in line with your right shoulder *(far right)*. Follow your elbow with your arm, extending it fully to stretch the right side of your chest *(below)*. Repeat at least once and then stretch your left side.

Place your right hand and forearm over your left shoulder and grasp your right elbow with your left hand. Push your elbow towards your left shoulder.

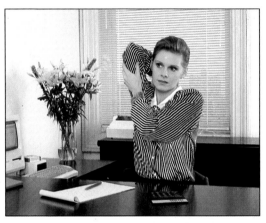

Bring your right hand over your right shoulder. Grasp your right elbow with your left hand and push your elbow backwards to stretch your upper arm.

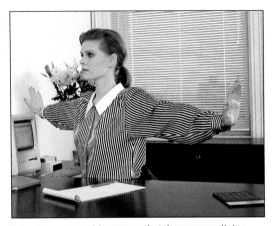

Extend your arms sideways so that they are parallel to the floor. Flex your hands so that your fingers point up and make circling motions with your hands and arms.

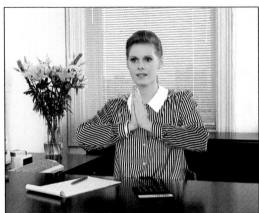

Place your palms together in front of you, fingers pointed up. Press your hands together hard for five seconds, then relax. Repeat three times.

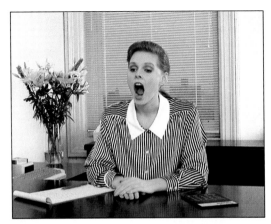

Rest your hands on your desk and look straight ahead. Drop your jaw and open your mouth as wide as you can. Keep your face relaxed.

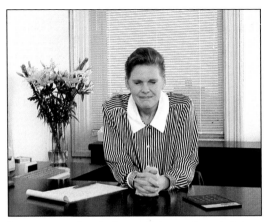

Close your mouth and grimace. Relax your jaws, but tighten your lips and shut your eyes. Alternate this exercise several times with the jaw opener on the left.

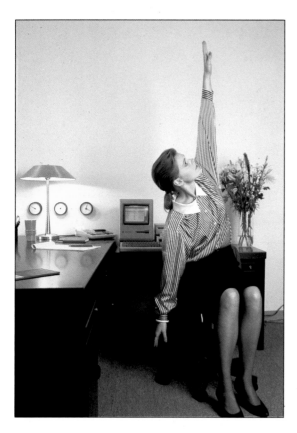

Turn your chair away from your desk and sit up straight. Drop your right hand towards the floor and extend your left hand towards the ceiling, stretching your entire left side. Repeat on your right side.

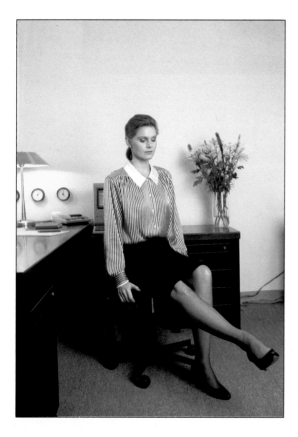

Brace yourself by holding the sides of your chair. Keeping your left foot flat on the floor, extend your right leg out parallel to the floor and flex your foot, stretching your hamstrings. Repeat for your left leg.

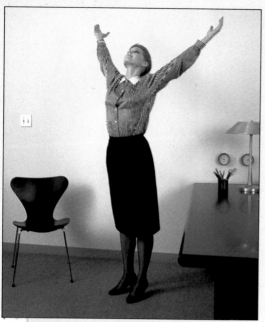

Stand up and take a deep breath. Tilt your head back and throw out your arms as if you were greeting the ceiling *(above)*. Exhale as you slowly relax your body, bending your knees slightly and dropping your hands to the floor *(below)*. Remain bent over for a few seconds before slowly taking a deep breath and returning to the greet-the-ceiling pose.

Hand Massage

The interlocking web of muscles, tendons and bones that makes up each of your hands is one of the body's most anatomically complex structures. Your hands must translate thought into action — whether it be the brute force of swinging an axe or lifting bales of hay, or the precise co-ordination of dialling a telephone number. The range of motion provided by the arms allows your hands to reach practically anywhere on your body.

Office work can be fatiguing for your hands, particularly if you use them throughout the day with little or no rest. Long hours of punching numbers on a calculator, typing or writing can produce stiffness and muscle spasm. You can prevent or relieve tension in your hands with this five-minute exercise and self-massage routine, which not only relaxes tight muscles, but strengthens them, too.

1. Place a tennis ball or a piece of foam in the palm of your hand. Grip and release the ball or foam. Repeat 12 times.

2. Put a rubber band around your fingers; open and close them at least 20 times. The thicker the band, the more difficult.

6. Continue pressing *(Step 5)*, slowly moving towards the space between the first two fingers. Repeat for each pair of fingers.

7. Turn your hand over and massage the back of the hand, starting at the base and working towards your fingertips.

3. Make loose fists with both your hands, then move your fists in a circle to increase your range of motion.

4. Pat or gently slap your hands all over, particularly on the back and the fingers. This helps to increase circulation.

5. Open one hand and grasp it with the other. Press the thumb firmly on the base of the hand for a second or two.

8. Grip the fleshy portion between your thumb and index finger. Press and release it at least five times.

9. Grip the knuckle of the thumb of one hand between the thumb and index finger of the other. Move the thumb in a circle.

10. Grasp your index finger and rotate it in a circular motion. Move each finger in a similar manner.

Lunchtime Aerobics/1

Aerobic exercise such as running, swimming or cycling is probably the most powerful anti-stress therapy you can practise. Although such exercises normally require you to be outdoors or in a pool, or to use special equipment, you can conveniently perform a good indoor aerobics routine — one that works your body's large muscles and raises your heart rate — during your lunch hour. Studies show that aerobics, when done properly, is also an effective way to relieve stress.

As with other aerobic routines, you should exercise at least three times a week for 30 minutes a session, with each session consisting of a five-minute warm-up, a 20-minute aerobic phase and a five-minute cool-down. During the aerobic phase, your heart rate should be somewhere between 65 and 85 per cent of your maximum heart rate. (Subtract your age from 220 to find your maximum heart rate. Then multiply this figure by 0.65 and also by 0.85 to calculate the boundaries of the target heart rate zone.)

Make a tape of music to fit the length of your session. Any type of music with a steady beat is suitable. Fit the tempo to the exercise — the music for the aerobic phase should be more lively than for the warm-up and cool-down.

To avoid injury, be sure to wear a good pair of aerobics shoes and try not to jump during any of the movements. In other words, keep one foot on the floor at all times.

For your warm-up, perform the five movements shown on these two pages for 30 seconds each, then repeat the entire sequence.

To begin the warm-up phase, ease your body into the routine by walking on the spot: swing your arms at your sides, and alternate rolling up and down from the heel to the ball of the foot.

Continue walking on the spot to the beat of the music. Rotate your left shoulder to increase its flexibility. Then rotate the right.

Once your shoulders are loosened up, bend your left elbow and circle it to the back. Then circle your right elbow back.

While you are still stepping to the beat of the music, rotate both your arms in large circles with your hands outstretched.

Pretend you are performing the breaststroke. Extend your arms in front of you, bend your elbows, then press your palms to the side and back, parallel to your shoulders. Bend your arms at the elbows again and return to the starting position.

Lunchtime Aerobics/2

The movements for the aerobic phase, shown here and on pages 74-75, are designed to increase the intensity of your session. To ensure that you are working in your training heart rate range, take your pulse every five minutes. Count the number of beats for 10 seconds and multiply by six. If your heart rate is below 65 per cent of its maximum *(see page 70)*, then you should work more vigorously. Repeat the routine for 20 minutes. If you have not been exercising for some time, start with five minutes and lengthen your workout by 10 per cent each week.

Jog on the spot and keep your arms raised. Interlace your fingers and invert your palms *(left)*. Then raise them up over your head *(top)*. Bring your arms down to chest level and extend them out to each side *(above)*. Repeat 10 times.

Jog on the spot and perform a rowing exercise and arm extension. Extend your arms and pull your hands back to your chest *(far left)*. Then extend your arms out to the sides *(left)*. Repeat 20 times.

While still jogging on the spot, bring your fists to your chest and then extend your left fist out to the side *(left)*. Return your left fist to your chest *(above)* before you fling your right fist to the side. Repeat 20 times for each arm.

Lunchtime
Aerobics/3

Alternately pump your arms above your head while kicking your legs from side to side for about two minutes *(right)*.

Run on the spot. Alternate flexing and extending your arms out to your sides, bringing your fists to your shoulders *(above)*. Then raise your arms above your head and make wide circles *(right)*.

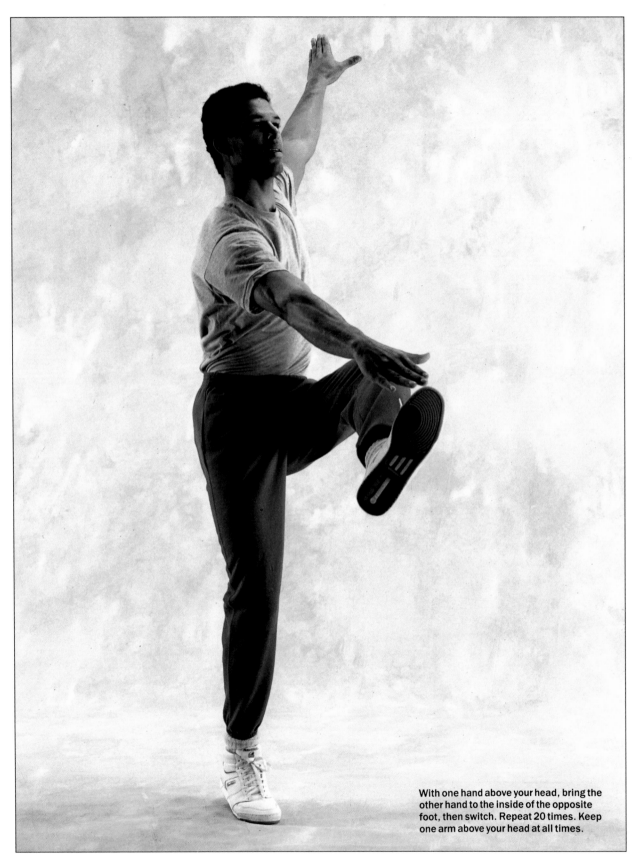

With one hand above your head, bring the other hand to the inside of the opposite foot, then switch. Repeat 20 times. Keep one arm above your head at all times.

Lunchtime Aerobics/4

After you have completed the aerobic portion of your workout, you should spend five minutes cooling down. If you stop your workout abruptly, you may experience a sudden drop in blood pressure, which can stress the heart. Cooling down lets your heart rate decelerate gradually and safely.

Many people use stretching routines as a warm-up for exercise. You will get the greatest benefit, however, if you stretch immediately *after* you have finished your routine. The stretches here are shown for one side of the body; be sure to repeat them on the other side. Hold each stretch for at least 20 seconds.

Stretch the muscles in your right side by bending your right knee and reaching up with your right arm *(above)*.

Bend at the waist and let your arms dangle *(above)*, keeping your weight centred over your toes. Flex your right knee slightly, while keeping your left leg straight, to stretch your left hamstrings and calf.

To cool down, jog on the spot, dropping your arms and swinging your legs to the side.

Lie on your back with your arms outstretched, your knees up and the soles of your feet flat on the floor. Keeping your arms on the floor, bring both knees to the left and turn your head to the right.

Draw your knees back up so that your feet are flat on the floor again. Cross your arms over your chest as if you were hugging yourself and bring your hands towards the floor.

Supporting yourself with your hands, sit straight up on the floor with your legs extended. Draw up your left foot and cross it over your right knee. Grasp your left knee with your right hand and pull back gently while you turn your trunk to the left.

Imaging

Focusing your mind on certain thoughts and images appears to reduce anxiety and help develop a state of relaxed alertness. As a technique for managing stress, a growing number of athletes perform imaging exercises before engaging in a demanding activity. A high jumper, for example, might stand at the approach to the bar, take a few deep breaths to clear his mind and eliminate all distractions, relax and concentrate intensely for a few moments. He visualizes himself in a complex series of movements: running down the approach in a certain number of steps, planting his feet, gathering his body up and lifting himself over the bar. Some athletes and coaches call this mental rehearsal the "inner game". When you visualize yourself performing, your mind and muscles stage a dress rehearsal in which low-level sequences of electrical impulses are actually sent to the muscles.

Mental imagery can be used to regulate not only physical performance, but also bodily responses. Some imaging techniques have been shown to affect the immune system and thus improve patients' chances of fighting cancer.

Imaging has also been shown to be an effective stress reducer. In a study of relaxation therapies for hypertensive patients, imaging was found to be as effective as a supervised stress-management programme in reducing blood pressure, during both treatment and follow-up.

To use imaging to reduce stress, find a comfortable chair in a quiet room free of distractions. Sit in the chair, close your eyes and breathe deeply, so that you are receptive to relaxation. Concentrate on a relaxing image. It does not matter what that image is as long as you can see yourself in that image and you associate it with deep relaxation.

Picture yourself on a tropical beach, for example. You can "see" the palm trees sway in the gentle breeze and "feel" the warmth of the sun on your forehead. Make the image as vivid as possible: you are wearing your favourite holiday shirt and shorts; the blue sea laps just a short distance from your toes. Seagulls circle over the water. Think not only of the visual images, but the sounds, tastes and scents as well.

While you think of your relaxing image, concentrate also on your own body as being relaxed and warm. Give yourself about 20 minutes per session to reduce tension.

Athletes routinely use imaging to prepare for demanding activities. Before attempting a difficult jump, for instance, a skier will rehearse the experience of jumping in his mind. Similarly, a pole vaulter *(inset)* will visualize his step-by-step approach to the high bar.

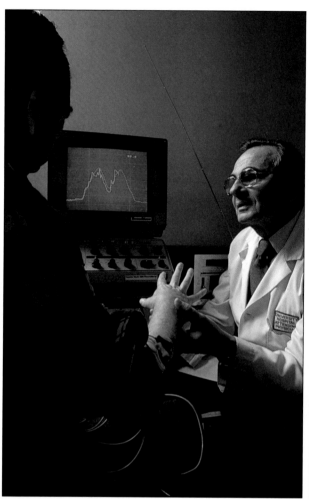

Biofeedback machines can measure such bodily functions as pulse rate, skin temperature and muscular tension. By monitoring a visual display, subjects can learn to control these functions.

Inexpensive, portable biofeedback machines can detect a single function, such as skin temperature or pulse rate in the fingertips, and relay that information by means of a tone.

Biofeedback

Most researchers and doctors believe that bodily functions controlled by the autonomic nervous system — such as heart rate and blood pressure — are involuntary. Regulation of these functions is normally carried on at a subconscious level and is therefore not directly governed by deliberate thought. However, when you can monitor these functions, it is possible to learn to control them consciously.

Subjects who are hooked up to biofeedback instruments can often be taught to recognize when they are tense and how to relax. Typically, a biofeedback machine reads minute changes in the skin's electrical conductivity, which gets stronger as muscle tension increases. If the machine determines that a subject is tense, it emits a tone. The subject is then told to make the tone go away by trying to relax mentally and physically. Through experimenting with different thoughts, images and breathing techniques, most people can make the tone decrease in volume and eventually disappear.

Researchers are not certain how biofeedback works. But they have determined that, by using biofeedback, subjects can consciously reduce their pulse rate and skin temperature. Biofeedback has also been found to be useful in helping some people overcome such stress-related symptoms as high blood pressure.

Researchers have also discovered that biofeedback can help control tinnitus, or ringing in the ears, a condition that many medical experts think is caused or aggravated by stress. In a study of 132 tinnitus patients who had not been helped by hypnosis, acupuncture, surgery, psychotherapy or drugs, 79 per cent reported that biofeedback gave relief in the duration, pitch or loudness of the attacks.

People who suffer from frequent stress-related tension headaches may benefit the most from biofeedback therapy. Biofeedback enables these patients to relax their muscles during stressful situations to prevent headaches from occurring and, when they already have a headache, to reduce the pain.

Biofeedback is usually a laboratory technique. However, a number of companies offer inexpensive biofeedback equipment for home use. You can also perform some simple biofeedback-imaging exercises without any equipment. Find a quiet room and sit in a comfortable chair. Close your eyes, take a few deep breaths and imagine that you are connected to a machine that controls your anxiety levels. To lower your stress and tension, slowly turn down the volume dial on the machine. As you adjust the dial, concentrate on your breathing and imagine that it is getting slower and deeper. Relax for 20 minutes using this technique.

A common site for measuring muscular tension is the forehead. Sensors detect the level of electrical charges in the muscles just below the skin.

REST

Another technique that can be used to induce relaxation is one that researchers refer to as restricted environmental stimulus therapy, or REST. Also known as sensory deprivation or sensory isolation, the technique usually involves floating in buoyant saline water kept at skin temperature in a soundproof and light-free chamber — a flotation tank — or lying on a bed in a similarly stimulus-free environment. Many studies have indicated that an hour or so in such an environment can produce deep relaxation, a sense of well-being and reduced pulse rate, blood pressure and feelings of anxiety. REST can also decrease muscular tension, particularly in the forehead, suggesting a possible treatment for tension headaches. In addition, both systolic and diastolic blood pressure decrease during REST treatment and follow-up in those who have hypertension as well as in those who do not.

When the body is free of outside stimuli, the production of many stress hormones has been shown to decrease. As with biofeedback, researchers have not yet determined exactly why REST brings about these effects. According to one theory, REST evokes the relaxation response by allowing the subject to become more aware of his or her internal processes. With this awareness comes an increased ability to focus on and control specific bodily functions, such as heart rate.

You do not need an expensive, stimulus-free flotation tank to achieve the desired result in a REST programme. One good way to relax is to float in a warm, calm pool. It helps to fill the pool with salt water, since you will be more buoyant than in fresh water. But you can also use a life jacket or another flotation device that allows you to float on your back without having to worry about keeping your mouth above water.

Lie face up in a pool with your arms and legs slightly outstretched. Do not tread water; instead, concentrate on becoming completely relaxed. Close your eyes. Breathe slowly and easily but do not take large, gulping breaths, since doing so will cause you to bob up and down. Clear your mind as much as possible and remain in this position for 15 to 20 minutes.

Pet Therapy

Until recently, the small amount of research on the interaction between pets and their owners concerned only diseases spread by animals and related health problems. Now there is evidence that pets can reduce stress, as pet owners have known for a long time. Caring for a pet, researchers theorize, can provide a sense of belonging, opportunities for play and entertainment.

Studies show that owning a pet — whether it be a dog or cat, bird or fish — can reduce the mild stress levels associated with minor, everyday frustrations. Animal ownership appears to be associated with improved health, lower blood pressure, reduced anxiety and at least a temporary reduction in stress levels. Even the presence of animals may have a calming effect in certain situations: in a study of children who were tested while at rest and while reading a poem aloud, those who were in a room with a friendly dog had lower blood-pressure levels and heart rates than those who were not.

Fish and other pets have proved effective when used as therapy, particularly in combating loneliness, in many institutions for the elderly, the handicapped and the mentally disturbed. In one study, inmates in a psychiatric hospital who were allowed to keep fish tanks in their wards engaged in fewer fights and made fewer suicide attempts.

An aquarium can calm you down. In a study of stress in dental patients, researchers found that patients who had a fish tank to look at in the waiting room showed significantly lower anxiety levels than those who had none. The aquarium was even more effective than hypnosis in allaying patients' fears.

CHAPTER FOUR

Evening

The stresses — and the comforts — of family and friends

Evening is a time for being with the family. Traditionally, the family has been viewed as a haven from stress, a buffer from the hardships, frustrations and injustices of the day. Although this view has been challenged in recent years, it is still commonly believed that the family is — and ought to be — a sort of life belt in a sea of stress.

Unfortunately, the family is not perfectly endowed to deal with stress; in fact, the family itself can be one of the most devastating sources of stress. Primary family stresses — those that are generated within the family — include such milestones as marriage, divorce, childbirth and the death of a parent or spouse. These events are so disruptive and intensely stressful that one or more of them can lead to stress-related illness or accidents.

Other forms of family-related stress identified by researchers are less immediately painful but can also be troublesome. The most common of these are role overload, when family and career obligations conflict; role underload, when a housewife, for instance, resents having to perform her designated role; and role captivity, when one partner feels trapped in his or her role.

These primary stresses can be compounded by secondary stresses, those generated outside the family, especially when the affected person wants to shield other family members from this stress. For instance, many people try to leave their on-the-job problems at work, but, more often than not, the attempt fails. Other family members notice a change in the behaviour of the stressed person and mistakenly assume they have caused that change, thus straining the relationship. In addition, when secondary stress is either pent up or misdirected, it often promotes or contributes to primary family stress, leading to a spiral of stress that may be difficult to deal with.

Stress can also take its toll on your sex life. Studies show that stress can lower sex hormone levels in the blood of both men and women, which may negatively affect sexual performance. If stress has eroded your sex life, the resulting unsatisfactory sex, or lack of sex, will also contribute to the stress spiral.

Talking about and sharing your anxieties is difficult for many people, but talking about specific problems — what psychologists call problem-focused coping — is usually the best way of dealing with the situation. Such difficulties as feeling powerless at work or resenting the unequal distribution of household chores should be addressed in specific terms, with the aim of pursuing realistic goals and finding solutions. Simply "cheering up" someone under stress can be soothing but may not be an effective way of relieving problems.

Although family life has many stresses, the view of marriage as a life belt does have validity. Many studies have noted, for instance, that mortality rates are significantly higher for single and divorced people than for those who are married. Studies show that those who are single and live alone have premature death rates from two to 10 times that of married people. Divorced white males, for instance, are more than twice as likely as married counterparts to die from heart disease, cirrhosis of the liver, hypertension and lung and stomach cancer. Single, divorced and widowed white women, too, have significantly higher mortality rates than their married counterparts.

Recent studies have also shown that a network of friends is a powerful bulwark against the stresses of life. Friends can provide many of the same benefits as family members, including emotional support during crises. Researchers have found that people who lack ties that provide intimacy, reassurance of worth and other emotional supports are particularly susceptible to stress-related illnesses.

Although you can enlist your friends, spouse and other family members to help you deal with your problems and anxieties, you can also

A Good Night's Sleep

A sound sleep can restore you both mentally and physically. Yet according to American surveys, between 15 and 20 per cent of the adult population routinely suffer from insomnia, a general term that refers to difficulty falling asleep or sleeping soundly. Chronic insomnia is often triggered by anxiety, but it may persist even after the source of stress is removed. If you have trouble getting to sleep, or if you do not regularly wake up feeling refreshed and alert, here are some suggestions:

◆ Establish a regular sleeping schedule, but do not try to force sleep. If you cannot fall asleep in 15 to 20 minutes, read until you feel drowsy. No matter when you fall asleep, always try to rise at the same time. Do not try to make up for lost sleep by taking naps or sleeping late at weekends.

◆ Do not drink coffee, tea, colas or any other caffeine-containing beverage within four hours of bedtime. Also, avoid alcohol and other drugs that will disrupt your sleep. And do not smoke before going to bed: nicotine can have a stimulating effect.

◆ At best, sleeping pills should be used only for occasional insomnia, and you should never take them for more than three nights in a row. These drugs can disrupt the body's natural sleep cycle and suppress the rapid eye movement (REM) sleep period, when dreams occur.

◆ Do not take your troubles to bed. Clear your mind and release your body's tensions through progressive-relaxation exercises like those on pages 116-117. For reading and sleeping positions that eliminate back stress, see pages 118-119.

benefit from setting aside time in the evening to deal with the cumulative effects of the day's stress. Often, the effects of generalized stress result in specific points of distress. You have an aching shoulder or back, for instance, although you have not been lifting heavy objects or otherwise straining your back. Or perhaps you notice that your jaws are clenched shut, even when you think you are relaxed, or that your partner complains that you kept him or her awake at night by grinding your teeth. All these are signs of stress that the exercises in this chapter, which are targeted to your symptoms, can relieve or prevent.

One of the best ways to relax is through Yoga, which has been practised for centuries as a means of achieving inner peace and relaxation. It is also the basis for most stretching exercises that relieve muscular tension, which often results from stress, and speed recovery from muscle strains and overuse injuries.

A much newer relaxation method is called progressive relaxation, in which you tense and relax various muscle groups in succession from head to toe. Progressive relaxation has been shown to reduce some types of headache, backache and other symptoms of stress and is an effective, convenient method of clearing your mind and releasing tension in your body as you prepare for bed. This chapter also shows you the proper posture for lying in bed, which can help relieve strain on the spine as well as prepare you for sleep.

Headache Intervention

Pressures and stresses that mount during the day often result in a headache. Although millions of people suffer chronic headaches severe enough for them to seek a remedy, medical science still does not fully understand these ailments. The most common types are vascular headaches, which include migraines, and tension headaches.

Vascular headaches result from the constriction or dilation of blood vessels in the brain. Migraines, which may be the most severe as well as the most long lasting, usually run in families and tend to strike more women than men.

Tension headaches, probably the most common form of headaches, are often caused by muscular contractions in the head and neck. Typically, patients report a dull, band-like pressure or pain in the forehead and the back of the head or neck. Massaging tight head and neck muscles can help prevent such headaches or relieve them.

If you get a tension headache, apply a compress by dampening a towel with either hot or cold water and wrapping it round your forehead or the back of your neck. This will help relax the muscles and prepare them for the headache-intervention massage routine which is described on these two pages.

Brace the fingers of one hand on your forehead. Press your thumb on the upper inside edge of the eye cavity.

Place your second finger on top of your index finger and firmly stroke along the region underneath your eyes.

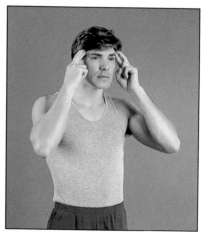

Press your fingers into the fleshy portion of your temples just above eye level. Massage in a circular motion.

Warm up the back of your scalp and increase the circulation to the skin by briskly massaging the area.

Drop your head, brace your fingers and, with your thumbs, firmly massage the back of your neck just below the skull.

With your head down, press your fingers into the fleshy portion of your neck on both sides of your spine. Massage up and down.

Place the fingertips of both hands in the centre of your forehead over the bridge of your nose. Press firmly and pull your hands apart across your forehead *(opposite)*.

Lower Back Pain Relief/1

About eight out of every 10 people suffer from lower back pain at one time or another. A smaller but still sizable fraction of the population endures chronic lower back pain, and in the worst cases some people are permanently disabled as a result. Yet in the majority of cases there is no discernible cause for all this misery.

Most lower back pain is preventable. More than 80 per cent of all such pain is muscular in nature and is at least an indirect result of muscle weakness, inflexibility and tension. Obesity is also a common factor in many cases of lower back pain.

Often, psychological stress that builds up for a long time manifests itself in muscle cramps in the back, particularly if you are predisposed to back pain for the reasons cited. Correct posture *(pages 60-61)* and sleeping positions *(pages 118-119)* may relieve lower back pain.

To prevent lower back pain, you should control your weight with a proper diet and aerobic exercise. You can also strengthen and stretch the appropriate muscles by performing the exercises described on this and the following three pages.

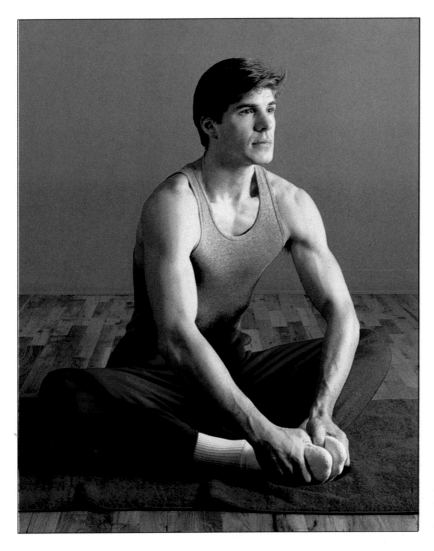

Sit on the floor and place the soles of your feet together. Grasp your feet and lean forwards from the hips, keeping your back as straight as possible. This will stretch your lower back and inner thigh muscles.

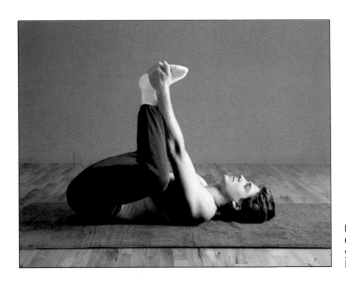

Lie on your back and draw your feet up. Grasp your feet and pull your knees towards your chest, stretching your lower back and hamstring muscles.

Perform the cat and the camel. Get on your hands and knees and arch your back, hollowing your stomach. Then relax and reverse the arch. Repeat 10 times.

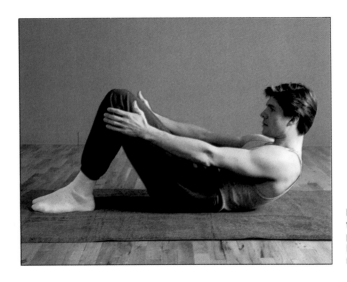

Lie on your back with your feet flat on the floor. Tighten your abdominal muscles and perform a partial sit-up, extending your hands next to your knees. Hold briefly and repeat at least five times.

Lower Back Pain Relief/2

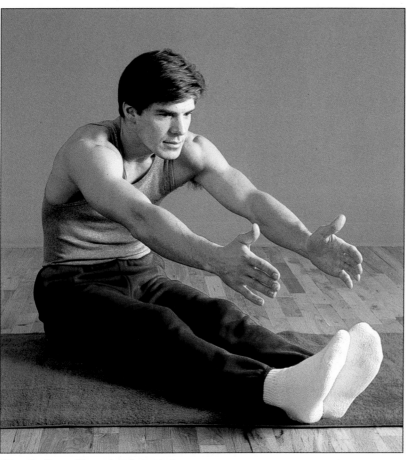

Sit on the floor with your legs extended
and your feet together. Flex your knees
slightly so that they do not lock. With your
back as straight as possible, lean forwards
and extend your hands over your feet. Hold
for 20 seconds to stretch your hamstrings.

To perform a lunge, prop your hands on
your left knee and lean forwards to stretch
your right hip flexors. Repeat to stretch
your left hip flexors.

To stretch your hip flexors, stand with your back to a stool and place your right foot on the seat. Bend your left knee and hold the position for at least 20 seconds to stretch your right hip flexors. Repeat with the right knee.

Back Massage

The relaxing effects that follow from a good back rub can be extremely pleasurable, and scientific evidence now confirms that a back massage can significantly reduce anxiety, lower the heart rate and lessen muscular tension. One study examined men and women with clinical symptoms of stress — including neck, shoulder and back pain, impaired peripheral circulation and poor sleep — who were still unable to relax after regular doses of muscle relaxants, anti-anxiety drugs and other standard medical treatments. In every subject studied, 30 to 45 minutes of back massage significantly and consistently reduced tension. Many of these individuals also reported profoundly refreshing sleep during the nights following the massage treatment, and most reduced or stopped their drug treatments after 10 or more sessions.

Even if you do not suffer clinical symptoms of stress, you can benefit from a relaxing back massage from a friend, a spouse or another family member. The only supplies you will need are a towel and a bottle of vegetable oil: spreading oil on your skin will facilitate the massage strokes. If you wish, you can buy a perfumed massage oil at a health food shop or other speciality shop. You should find a room with a carpet, or else provide a towel or a piece of foam to cover the floor.

Lie face down on the floor with your hands at your sides *(opposite)*. Your partner kneels by your head and fans her fingers out over your back. She then leans forwards to provide maximum pressure and pushes her hands down to the small of your back on either side of your spine. She draws her hands up your back, away from your spine, to your neck. Repeating the motion at least three times, your partner traces a heart shape each time, with the point of the heart at the nape of your neck.

Turn your face to the right. Your partner grasps your head with one hand and your left shoulder with the other. She presses her hands in opposite directions and holds a stretch for 10 seconds.

Remain in a prone position as your partner kneads your shoulder muscles with her thumbs, pressing firmly in a circular motion until you feel a release of muscular tightness or tension.

Stay face down on the floor as your partner kneels over your head. She leans over, using her body weight to apply pressure as she "walks" down the sides of your spine with her thumbs.

Foot Massage

Your feet routinely sustain a tremendous amount of stress. With every stride, they must conform to the contours of the ground, keep your body balanced and propel you forwards. All the while they must absorb shock — from 120 per cent of your body weight with each walking step to more than five times your body weight for each sprinting stride.

That the foot can readily absorb these stresses is clearly a marvel of biomechanical engineering. Still, the muscles, tendons and ligaments sup-ported by the 26 small bones in each foot can become fatigued by in-appropriate or ill-fitting foot gear or by the pressures of excessive stand-ing, walking, running or jumping. A good foot massage can help to reduce soreness, swelling and mus-cular tension, improve circulation, speed healing and restore range of motion to injured areas of the foot.

Muscle soreness in the feet can have several different causes. One possible cause is the build-up of lactic acid and other metabolic by-products, which accumulate in over-worked muscles. These by-products may irritate nerve endings and cause muscle contraction and pain. A sec-ond cause is minutely torn tissue, which results from unaccustomed work and fatigue. Another cause of sore or inflamed feet may be connective-tissue irritation.

Foot massage can help reduce the symptoms of soreness by encourag-ing circulation and lymph flow, removing metabolic wastes and relaxing muscles. After massaging one foot, perform the routine shown here on the other foot.

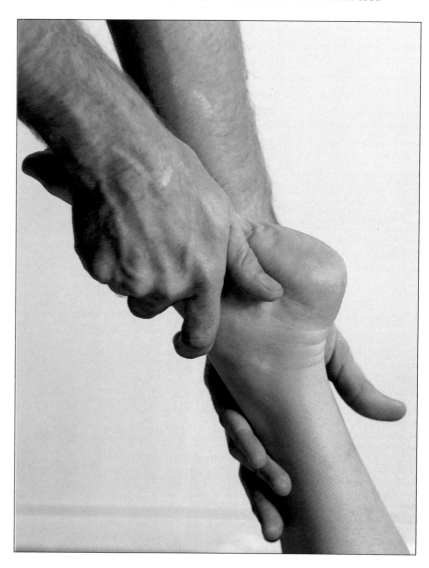

Gentle stroking is a good warm-up for the foot to prepare it for more intensive massage. Lie face down and bend one knee. Your partner stands behind you and slowly but firmly strokes one foot, alternately pulling from the bottom of the shin to the end of the toes with each hand.

Your partner presses on the ball of your foot and massages your Achilles tendon.

From the heel to the ball of your foot, he presses deeply with a rotary thumb motion.

For soothing traction of your toe joints, your partner pulls gently on each toe.

His thumb presses into the intermetatarsal spaces between the bones in your midfoot.

Turn over so that your partner can grasp your ankle and push your foot up and down.

He then presses his thumb into the spaces between the bones on the top of your toes.

Facial Massage

The body's most complex latticework of muscles and tendons is in the face. No fewer than 69 muscles control the nearly infinite variety of expressions you display daily. Since your facial muscles are so sensitively tuned to your emotions and state of mind, your face involuntarily reflects your joy, amusement and surprise, as well as anxiety, stress and pain. Emotional tension, for instance, can often be measured by electromyographic tracings of neural activity in facial muscles. But the face does not just serve as a mirror of your emotions; it can also govern them to some extent. Studies have shown that some individuals learn to unwind simply by concentrating on relaxing their forehead muscles.

You can reduce facial tension without isolating and relaxing specific muscles. Just let a relaxing facial massage do the work for you. Facial massage can reduce muscular tension in the forehead, round the eyes, in the jaw area and even in the neck — areas where stress often causes tightness and pain.

Your face is bonier and less fragile than it may seem, so your partner can apply forceful massage without causing discomfort. Be sure to instruct your partner, however. Let him know how hard to press, especially at the beginning, so that you get an effective massage without undue discomfort.

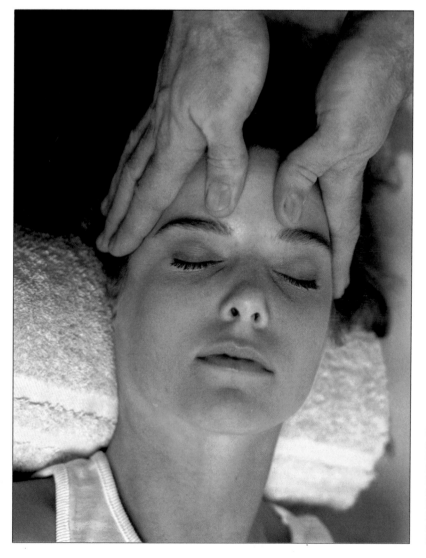

Lie on your back with your head resting securely on a pillow or towel. Your partner kneels over your head and presses his thumbs firmly on to the top of your forehead near your hairline. He then pulls his thumbs apart along the hairline by letting his hands glide down the side of your head. He repeats the process several times, moving his thumbs progressively closer to your eyebrows *(left)*.

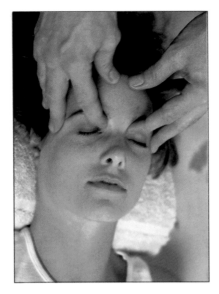

Your partner rest his thumbs on your forehead and makes gentle circular motions on the upper part of your eye sockets with his index finger.

Next, he places the heels of his hands on either side of your nose and presses firmly, gliding his hands slowly down your cheeks towards your jaws.

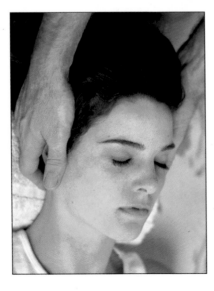

Completing the cheek push, your partner slides his hands under the back of your neck and up your skull, pulling back and up to give you gentle, relaxing neck traction. He then repeats the facial massage.

Jaw Unclenchers

Bruxism, or unconscious clenching and grinding of the teeth, is a very common affliction. Also called TMJ syndrome, after the temporomandibular or jaw joint, bruxism can result in worn and displaced teeth, toothache, pain in the jaw, ear or neck, tension headache and dysfunction of the temporomandibular joint.

Tension-related stress that triggers jaw-muscle spasms can be a cause of bruxism. The jaw relaxers on these two pages will help alleviate it.

Hold a cork between your teeth for several minutes. To avoid overstretched muscles, be sure you can open your mouth 5 mm more than the length of the cork.

Open your mouth as wide as possible. Use your whole face to stretch your jaw muscles. You can even roll your eyes and stick out your tongue.

With your mouth open wide, try to move your lower jaw to the right to stretch the muscles that grind your teeth together from one side to the other.

Open your mouth once again and try to move your lower jaw to the left as far as possible. Close your eyes and scrunch up your face to increase the effort.

The lion position, a Yoga posture, can help to relax your facial muscles. Sit in the lotus position or cross-legged on the floor *(opposite)*. Extend your arms and place your palms on your knees. Keep your eyes wide open, extend your tongue and exhale, like a lion, with a breathy rasp.

Yoga/1

Drawing a quiet breath, calming the mind and soothing the body are the essence of relaxation. They are also the soul of Yoga. Instructors of Hatha Yoga, one of several Yoga disciplines, teach stretching positions — the lotus *(page 52)* is perhaps the most familiar — and controlled breathing.

Studies that have been conducted on the physiological effects of Yoga yield conflicting results. Some studies report more rapid heart rates, higher blood pressure, faster respiration and greater oxygen consumption during yogic meditation; others report precisely the opposite findings. Strangely, almost all the studies that took electroencephalograph (EEG) measurements of those practising Yoga showed a reduction of alpha-brainwave activity. Furthermore, the EEGs were not affected by outside stimuli, such as flashing lights or noises. This suggests that those who practise Yoga and meditation can shut out external influences.

Recent studies by Indian medical researchers show that Yoga can provide relief from a variety of stress-related diseases and conditions, including hypertension, heart attack, peptic ulcer, insomnia and drug addiction. One unorthodox test showed that rats that had been annoyed by electrical pulses became calm and relaxed when held in Yoga positions.

The photographs on these two and the following 10 pages depict Yoga stretches and postures that involve standing, sitting, kneeling and lying down. Take your time when performing the exercises; breathe normally but slowly.

Stand or sit erect and draw your shoulders up as high as they can go *(top)*. Then abruptly release your shoulders and let them drop freely *(above)*.

Remain standing or seated in the same relaxed position and roll your eyes towards the ceiling *(top)*. Move your eyes round in a clockwise direction *(above)*.

Stand or sit erect and slowly turn your head to the left *(opposite)*. Hold for at least 20 seconds. Then drop your left ear towards your shoulder *(inset)* and hold. Repeat both exercises, turning your head to the right.

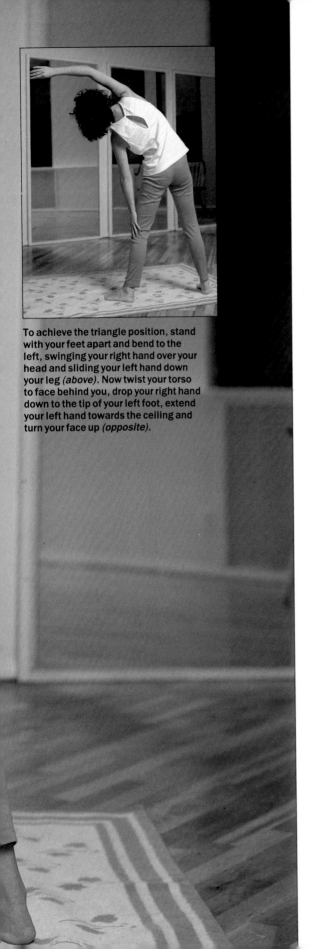

To achieve the triangle position, stand with your feet apart and bend to the left, swinging your right hand over your head and sliding your left hand down your leg *(above)*. Now twist your torso to face behind you, drop your right hand down to the tip of your left foot, extend your left hand towards the ceiling and turn your face up *(opposite)*.

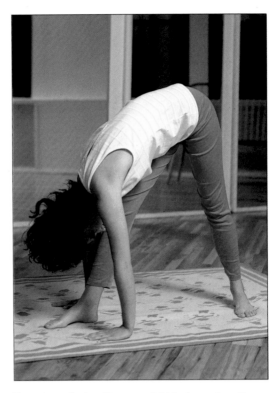

Spread your feet and turn your right foot away from the left. Twist to the right. Set your palms on the floor on both sides of your foot. Bend your right knee slightly.

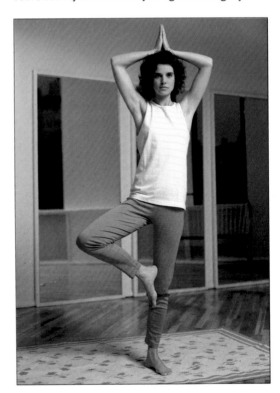

Assume the relaxing tree stance by standing erect and resting your right foot on the inside of your left leg. Put your palms together and rest them on your head.

107

Sit on the floor and draw your knees up *(right)*. Keep your lower legs and arms parallel to the floor. Hold this position for at least 20 seconds. For a more challenging exercise — which could strain your back if your abdominal muscles are not already well developed by such exercises as the one on the right — sit on the floor with your legs extended straight out and your hands on the floor at your sides for support. Slowly raise your legs, reclining slightly and balancing on your buttocks. Extend your arms straight out *(above)*.

Yoga/4

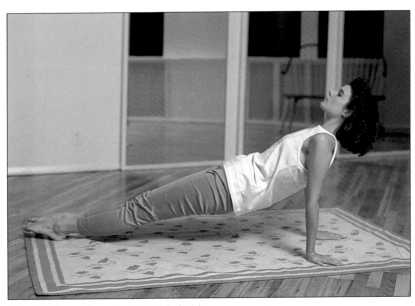

Sit on the floor with your legs extended and
your feet together. Support yourself on your
hands and raise your pelvis off the ground
so that your head, chest and pelvis form a
straight line down to your toes. Hold this
position for at least 20 seconds.

Sit on the floor with your legs extended and
opened wide. Keeping your back erect, turn
to your left; place your hands on the floor
for support. Repeat by turning to the right.

Begin the Yoga camel by kneeling on the floor and sitting on your heels *(opposite, inset)*. Place your hands on your heels, rise up on your knees, lift your chest towards the ceiling and press your hips forwards *(opposite)*. For an easier variation, lie on your back and place your feet flat on the floor so that you can grasp your heels. Press your hips towards the ceiling *(right)*.

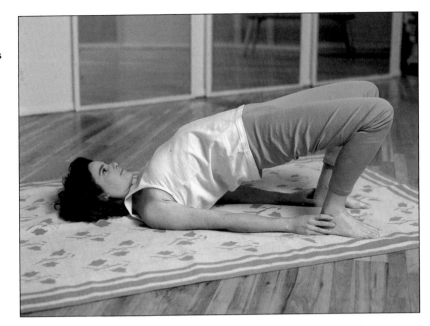

To perform the plough safely, lie on your back with your arms at your sides. Slowly swing your legs up over your head and place your toes on a pile of books. Be sure that your shoulders and arms, not your neck, support most of your body weight.

Lie on your back and draw your knees up. Grasp your upper shins and pull your knees towards your chest *(above)*. Extend your legs, holding on to your ankles so that your body forms a triangle *(below)*.

Yoga/6

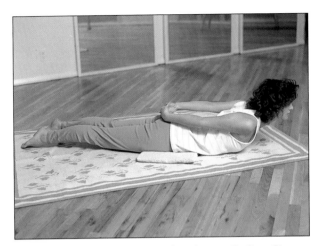

Fold a towel under your hips and lie face down on the floor. Place your arms at your sides and extend your toes. Bring your hands together behind your back and lift your chest and head.

Remain face down on the floor and extend your arms out in front of you. Lift your face, chest, arms and legs off the floor. Keep your arms parallel to the floor and your knees straight.

Bring your arms to your sides and make fists. Press your fists against the floor while lifting your head, chest and right leg, keeping your knee straight. Repeat for your left leg.

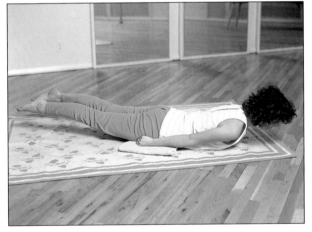

For the locust position, repeat the exercise on the left but lift both feet off the floor while pressing down with your fists. Make sure that your toes are extended and your knees are straight.

Progressive Relaxation

Progressive relaxation is a relatively new stress-reduction technique that involves systematically tensing and then relaxing most of the major muscles in the body. Tests show that people who practise progressive relaxation can significantly reduce their skin-temperature response and muscle tenseness, two measurements that scientists use to assess stress levels. In addition, progressive relaxation appears to be an effective therapy for certain stress symptoms, including migraine and tension headaches, hypertension, general anxiety and insomnia. Its effects can extend beyond the period when you are practising the technique: in some studies, subjects have been shown to remain in a relaxed state for several hours after each session. Other research has found that some patients on drug therapy for stress-related symptoms can reduce or discontinue their prescribed medication if they practise progressive relaxation.

You can obtain the calming benefits of progressive relaxation in just 10 to 20 minutes. First, find a room where you will not be disturbed by telephone calls or other interruptions and then take off your shoes. Wear comfortable, loose-fitting clothes.

Lie face up on a carpet or mat with your arms at your sides and your palms up *(right)*. Take a deep breath, hold it momentarily and then slowly exhale, thinking of the word "relax". Tighten your facial muscles as much as you can and hold this expression for five seconds *(inset, left)*. Relax. Tighten the muscles in your shoulders, your arms and then your hands *(inset, centre)*. Systematically move down your body, tightening and relaxing your muscles, concluding with your toes *(inset, right)*. Finally, lie still, breathe slowly and, employing mental imaging, think of a peaceful scene.

Sleep Positions

Although you have little control over the positions you assume while you sleep, you can control your position as you fall asleep. If you fall asleep in a relaxed position, you are more likely to enjoy a serene, refreshing rest.

First, it is important to have the right mattress. A mattress that is too soft will allow your torso to sink lower than the rest of your body, placing stress on your spine. On the other hand, a mattress that is too hard will make sleeping on your side uncomfortable.

Generally, lying on your stomach is not restful; it twists the neck and may stress the spine. Lying on your back is better, but often an excessively large pillow causes neck strain.

Although it is generally agreed that regular exercise promotes sound sleep, do not engage in a strenuous workout near bedtime. Quiet, contemplative exercises such as Yoga *(pages 104-115)* can improve your fitness without charging you up.

If you suffer lower back pain when you wake, go to sleep on your back with a pillow under your knees and a support under your neck.

For the most restful sleeping position, lie on your side with your neck and spine straight and your knees and elbows bent.

If reading is a way for you to relax before going to sleep, be sure to avoid strain by supporting your neck and spine adequately. The most restful position is to sit up in bed with pillows fully supporting your back, neck and head.

CHAPTER FIVE

B Vitamins

*Vital for healthy nerve cells,
release of energy from carbohydrates
and recovery from physical stress*

Vitamins are organic substances the body needs in minute amounts for growth and maintenance. Your body cannot manufacture vitamins, so food must supply them. Scientists categorize vitamins according to whether they are soluble in fat or in water; B vitamins (along with vitamin C) are water soluble. Except for B_{12}, none of the water-soluble vitamins can be stored in the body. Because they are constantly used up or excreted, you must consume adequate amounts of water-soluble vitamins frequently. On the other hand, fat-soluble vitamins (A, D, E and K) can be stored for relatively long periods and do not have to be consumed as often.

The eight vitamins known collectively as the B complex are B_1 (thiamine), B_2 (riboflavin), B_3 (niacin), B_5 (pantothenic acid), B_6 (pyridoxine), B_{12} (cyanocobalamin), folacin (or folic acid) and biotin. The sudden popularity of so-called stress vitamins, which contain large amounts of the B complex, arises from the fact that a diet lacking in some B vitamins may cause problems for someone recovering from

121

physical stress, such as burns or broken bones. However, chronic deficiencies of B complex vitamins are rare in Western countries, and no scientific evidence supports the claim that taking B vitamins in excess of the Recommended Daily Amount (RDA) helps you to cope with psychological stress.

In certain conditions where physical stress occurs, supplements may be advisable. B complex vitamins are sometimes prescribed for patients recovering from surgery. Some studies indicate that asthmatics may need supplementary doses of vitamin B_6. And vegans may need to supplement their diets with B_{12}: a serious deficiency of B_{12}, an important nutrient which is found only in foods of animal origin, prevents the normal development of red blood cells and can result in pernicious anaemia.

Although vitamins are not energy sources, several B vitamins play crucial roles in converting carbohydrates into glucose, a simple sugar that the body "burns" to provide energy, and in the metabolism of protein and fats. The B complex is also necessary for the working of the central nervous system, the synthesis of genetic material and a host of other bodily functions.

The B complex is distributed in a wide variety of foods, and a balanced diet supplies all you need of these vitamins. Weight for weight, brewer's yeast is the single richest source of B vitamins. Liver and other organ meats also supply abundant amounts. Milk, eggs, poultry and lean meat provide many B vitamins; pork is particularly rich in thiamine and niacin. Other good sources include whole-grain breads and cereals, brown rice, beans, peas and nuts. In Britain, white flour, breakfast cereals and other grain products made from processed wheat are enriched to replace some of their lost thiamine, niacin and iron. But other B vitamins lost in processing, as well as fibre and vitamin E, are not replaced, which is why enriched white flour is less nutritious than whole-grain flour.

There are Recommended Daily Amounts for three of the eight B vitamins. The adult requirement for thiamine is 1.0 to 1.3 milligrams; riboflavin, 1.3 to 1.6 milligrams; niacin, 15 to 18 milligrams. In addition, most nutritionists agree that you need about 2 milligrams of vitamin B_6, 200 micrograms of folacin and 3 micrograms of vitamin B_{12} a day. One tablespoon of brewer's yeast supplies from 25 to 100 per cent of the recommended amounts of most B vitamins. Ninety grams of beef liver provides 20 to 100 per cent of your daily need for all B vitamins, including enough B_{12} to last nearly a month.

If you exercise regularly, you need an increased intake of thiamine to metabolize the extra food that exercising demands. One recent study found that women who exercise may need more riboflavin than inactive women because of their increased energy output. You can easily satisfy this greater need by eating complex carbohydrates, such as those in whole grains, as well as low-fat dairy products and small amounts of organ meats. Although some athletes claim that B

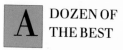

A DOZEN OF THE BEST

The following foods are all high in B complex vitamins.

MEAT AND DAIRY SOURCES:
Beef
Chicken
Eggs
Liver
Milk (and other dairy foods)
Pork

NON-MEAT SOURCES:
Brewer's yeast
Dark green leafy vegetables
Peas
Hazelnuts
Wheat germ
Whole grains

The Basic Guidelines

For a moderately active adult, Britain's National Advisory Committee on Nutrition Education recommends a diet that is low in fat, high in carbohydrates and moderate in protein. The committee's proposals for the long term suggest that no more than 30 per cent of your calories come from fat, that around 11 per cent come from protein and hence that 55 to 60 per cent come from carbohydrates. A gram of fat equals nine calories, while a gram of protein or carbohydrate equals four calories; therefore, if you eat 2,100 calories a day, you should consume approximately 70 grams of fat, 310 grams of carbohydrate and 60 grams of protein daily. If you follow a low-fat/high-carbohydrate diet, your chance of developing heart disease, cancer and other life-threatening diseases may be considerably reduced.

◆ The nutrition charts that accompany each of the low-fat/high-carbohydrate recipes in this book include the number of calories per serving, the number of grams of fat, carbohydrate and protein in a serving, and the percentage of calories derived from each of these nutrients. In addition, the charts provide the amount of calcium, iron and sodium per serving.

◆ Calcium deficiency may be associated with periodontal diseases — which attack the mouth's bones and tissues, including the gums — in both men and women, and with osteoporosis, or bone shrinking and weakening, in elderly women. The deficiency may also contribute to high blood pressure. The daily allowance for calcium recommended by the United Kingdom Department of Health and Social Security (DHSS) is 500 milligrams a day for men and women. Pregnant and lactating women are advised to consume 1,200 milligrams daily.

◆ Although one way you can reduce your fat intake is to cut your consumption of red meat, you should make sure that you get your necessary iron from other sources. The DHSS suggests a minimum of 10 milligrams of iron per day for men and 12 milligrams for women between the ages of 18 and 54.

◆ High sodium intake is associated with high blood pressure in susceptible people. Most adults should restrict sodium intake to about 2,000 milligrams a day, according to the World Health Organization. One way to keep sodium consumption in check is not to add table salt to food.

vitamin supplements enhance performance or endurance, no scientific study supports that claim.

When foods are processed or carelessly stored or prepared, large amounts of their B vitamins can be destroyed or lost. Milk stored in glass bottles and exposed to direct sunlight or fluorescent light, for example, can lose most of its riboflavin in three and a half hours.

The recipes that follow feature healthy ingredients that not only are rich in B vitamins, but are prepared in ways that minimize vitamin loss. Few recipes supply all of the B vitamins, so you should always eat a varied diet. Besides being rich in B vitamins, liver and other organ meats are high in cholesterol. Therefore, they are used in small portions in these recipes and combined with other foods rich in B vitamins, such as wheat germ, potatoes, beans and whole grains.

Breakfast

FRIED OATMEAL

Oats contain vitamin E as well as all of the B vitamins except B$_{12}$. Rolled oats are a whole grain, and research suggests that the water-soluble fibre in oats can help hold down blood cholesterol levels.

45 g (1½ oz) rolled oats	**1 teaspoon unsalted butter**
3 tablespoons raisins	**2 teaspoons plain flour**
2 teaspoons sugar	**¼ teaspoon ground cinnamon**
1 teaspoon corn oil	**4 teaspoons pure maple syrup**

Combine the oats with 50 cl (16 fl oz) of water in a small saucepan and cook, uncovered, over low heat for about 45 minutes, or until the oats are soft and the liquid is almost totally absorbed. Add the raisins and sugar and cook for 1 minute, then increase the heat to high and cook, stirring, for 1 minute, or until any excess liquid evaporates. Spread the oatmeal in a thin layer in a 22 by 12 cm (9 by 5 inch) loaf tin and smooth the top with a spatula. Lay a sheet of plastic film on the surface of the oatmeal and refrigerate for at least 2 hours, or until firm. (The oatmeal can be prepared the night before.)

Using a metal spatula, loosen the edges of the oatmeal and turn it out on to a plate. Cut the sheet of oatmeal in half lengthwise, then crosswise to make four equal pieces. Heat the oil in a non-stick frying pan over medium heat. When the oil is hot, add the butter. When the butter melts, dust the oatmeal slices with the flour and cook them for about 2 minutes on each side, or until well browned. Place the slices on two plates, sprinkle with cinnamon and dribble each serving with 2 teaspoons of maple syrup.   Makes 2 servings

CALORIES per serving	175
71% Carbohydrate	32 g
4% Protein	2 g
25% Fat	5 g
CALCIUM	26 mg
IRON	1 mg
SODIUM	4 mg

MILLET PORRIDGE WITH APRICOTS

Unsulphured dried fruits retain more of their B vitamins than the sulphured varieties. Millet provides a good amount of protein as well as B vitamins.

25 cl (8 fl oz) apple juice	**75 g (2½ oz) unsulphured dried**
12.5 cl (4 fl oz) skimmed milk	**apricots, coarsely chopped**
¾ teaspoon grated lemon rind	**2 tablespoons desiccated**
½ teaspoon salt	**coconut**
100 g (3½ oz) millet	**15 g (½ oz) butter**

Combine the apple juice, milk and 35 cl (12 fl oz) of water in a medium-sized non-reactive saucepan and bring to the boil over medium-high heat. Add the lemon rind and salt, then slowly stir in the millet. Cover the pan, reduce the heat to low and simmer for 20 minutes. Add the apricots and coconut and cook, covered, for another 20 minutes, or until the millet is creamy, adding more water if all of the water evaporates before the millet is cooked. Remove the pan from the heat, stir in the butter and serve.   Makes 4 servings

CALORIES per serving	195
70% Carbohydrate	36 g
8% Protein	4 g
22% Fat	5 g
CALCIUM	58 mg
IRON	3 mg
SODIUM	323 mg

Wheat Waffles with Fruit Sauce

WHEAT WAFFLES WITH FRUIT SAUCE

One serving of these waffles contains more than 20 per cent of your daily allowance of thiamine, which your body needs for burning carbohydrates.

CALORIES per serving	420
58% Carbohydrate	64 g
12% Protein	-12 g
30% Fat	15 g
CALCIUM	236 mg
IRON	3 mg
SODIUM	284 mg

Fruit Sauce:

150 g (5 oz) peeled fresh
   pineapple, diced
75 g (2½ oz) unsulphured dried
   apricots, cut into 5 mm (¼ inch)
   strips
75 g (2½ oz) sultanas
1 cinnamon stick
1 teaspoon grated lime rind
2 tablespoons pure maple syrup

Waffles:

125 g (4 oz) wholemeal flour
150 g (5 oz) plain flour
4 tablespoons wheat germ
1 tablespoon baking powder
35 cl (12 fl oz) semi-skimmed milk
3 large eggs, separated
60 g (2 oz) unsalted butter, melted
1 tablespoon honey
45 g (1½ oz) desiccated coconut

Stir together the fruit, cinnamon stick, lime rind and 17.5 cl (6 fl oz) of water in a small non-reactive saucepan. Cover and bring to the boil, then reduce the heat and simmer, stirring occasionally, for 30 minutes. Stir in the maple syrup.

While the sauce is cooking, stir together the dry ingredients in a large bowl. In a medium-sized bowl, whisk together the milk, egg yolks, 45 g (1½ oz) of the butter and the honey until smooth. Add this mixture to the dry ingredients and stir just until blended. In another large bowl, using an electric mixer, beat the egg whites until stiff peaks form. Stir one quarter of the whites into the batter, then gently fold in the remaining whites. Preheat a waffle iron and brush it lightly with some of the remaining butter. Pour in about 12.5 cl (4 fl oz) of batter and bake for 2 to 3 minutes or according to the manufacturer's directions, until the waffle is browned and crisp. Make another five waffles in the same fashion, brushing the waffle iron with the remaining butter as necessary. Divide the waffles among six plates, top with the fruit sauce and sprinkle with the coconut.

Makes 6 servings

SUNRISE BREAKFAST DRINK

Bananas contain a substantial amount of potassium and some vitamin C. Instead of discarding overripe bananas, peel them, wrap them in foil and freeze them for making this drink.

CALORIES per serving	190
73% Carbohydrate	36 g
18% Protein	9 g
9% Fat	2 g
CALCIUM	230 mg
IRON	Trace
SODIUM	220 mg

35 cl (12 fl oz) buttermilk
4 tablespoons frozen orange juice concentrate

1 egg white
1 frozen banana, cut into chunks
2 orange slices for garnish

Combine the buttermilk, orange juice concentrate, egg white and banana in a blender and process until smooth and creamy. Pour the mixture into two glasses and garnish each with an orange slice.   Makes 2 servings

PRUNE-ORANGE SPREAD ON TOAST

This spread, a good alternative to jams and marmalade, contains few calories because it is made without any added sweetener.

CALORIES per serving	130
75% Carbohydrate	25 g
18% Protein	6 g
7% Fat	1 g
CALCIUM	48 mg
IRON	Trace
SODIUM	248 mg

10 stoned prunes
12.5 cl (4 fl oz) orange juice
½ teaspoon pure vanilla extract

165 g (5½ oz) low-fat cottage cheese (1% fat)
6 slices cracked-wheat bread

Place the prunes, orange juice and vanilla extract in a small non-reactive saucepan and cook, covered, over medium heat for about 15 minutes, or until the prunes are tender. Transfer the prunes and liquid to a food processor or blender and process until puréed. Add the low-fat cottage cheese and process the mixture until smooth. Toast the bread and spread some of the prune mixture on each slice.   Makes 6 servings

BREAKFAST PARFAIT

In addition to containing B vitamins, this satisfying dish is high in fibre.

CALORIES per serving	260
81% Carbohydrate	56 g
15% Protein	11 g
4% Fat	1 g
CALCIUM	71 mg
IRON	2 mg
SODIUM	235 mg

1 recipe quantity Prune-Orange Spread (above)
45 g (1½ oz) bite-sized shredded wheat

75 g (2½ oz) raisins

In three parfait glasses or wineglasses, layer the prune spread alternately with the shredded wheat and raisins. Or simply stir the prune spread, cereal and raisins together in three small bowls. Serve immediately.   Makes 3 servings

Lunch

CHICK-PEA PURÉE IN A PITTA POCKET

This sandwich provides about one fifth of the adult Recommended Daily
Amount of niacin, most of which comes from the wholemeal pitta bread.

2 garlic cloves
150 g (5 oz) canned chick-peas,
   rinsed and drained, ½ teaspoon of
   the liquid reserved
1 teaspoon lemon juice
1 teaspoon corn oil
½ teaspoon sesame oil

One 15 cm (6 inch) wholemeal
   pitta bread
30 g (1 oz) lettuce, shredded
1 small tomato, diced
5 small black olives, stoned and
   halved

CALORIES per serving	560
61% Carbohydrate	89 g
16% Protein	23 g
23% Fat	15 g
CALCIUM	185 mg
IRON	8 mg
SODIUM	789 mg

Blanch the garlic in boiling water for 4 minutes. Drain the garlic, cool under cold water and discard the peels. Combine the garlic, the chick-peas and reserved liquid, the lemon juice and oils in a food processor or blender and process until puréed. Halve the pitta and fill the halves with the chick-pea purée, lettuce, tomato and olives.   Makes 1 serving

Chick-Pea Purée in a Pitta Pocket

BAKED SHELLS VENETIAN STYLE

The liver in this recipe supplies about half of your daily need for thiamine and riboflavin and more than one third of your niacin requirement.

30 g (1 oz) butter or margarine
250 g (8 oz) onion, finely chopped
½ teaspoon dried tarragon, crumbled
2 chicken livers, trimmed and finely chopped (about 90 g/3 oz)
3 tablespoons flour
50 cl (16 fl oz) skimmed milk

90 g (3 oz) low-fat mozzarella, grated
½ teaspoon salt
¼ teaspoon white pepper
Pinch of grated nutmeg
250 g (8 oz) large shell pasta, cooked and drained
150 g (5 oz) frozen peas, thawed
4 tablespoons dry breadcrumbs

Preheat the oven to 180°C (350°F or Mark 4). Melt the butter in a medium-sized saucepan over medium heat. Stir in the onion and tarragon and sauté for about 3 minutes, or until the onion is softened. Add the livers and cook for 2 minutes. Add the flour and cook, stirring, for 1 minute. Add the milk and cook, whisking constantly, for 5 minutes. Stir in the mozzarella and cook, stirring occasionally, for 3 minutes, or until the cheese melts. Stir in the salt, pepper and grated nutmeg. Transfer the sauce to a large bowl, add the pasta and peas and toss until well combined. Spoon half of the mixture into a 1.5 litre (2½ pint) casserole and sprinkle with 2 tablespoons of the breadcrumbs. Top with the remaining pasta and breadcrumbs and bake for 25 to 30 minutes, or until the top is golden.   Makes 4 servings

CALORIES per serving	470
57% Carbohydrate	67 g
21% Protein	24 g
22% Fat	11 g
CALCIUM	339 mg
IRON	5 mg
SODIUM	608 mg

AUBERGINE-TOFU CASSEROLE

Tofu adds body and texture, as well as protein and B vitamins, to tuna, meat, pasta or vegetable casseroles.

750 g (1½ lb) aubergines
125 g (4 oz) sweet red pepper, chopped
250 g (8 oz) onion, finely chopped
2 garlic cloves, crushed
½ teaspoon sesame oil
150 g (5 oz) firm tofu, squeezed dry and mashed
60 g (2 oz) Edam cheese, grated

3 tablespoons grated Parmesan
90 g (3 oz) fresh wholemeal breadcrumbs
4 tablespoons chopped parsley
¼ teaspoon each salt, ground cumin and ground coriander
⅛ teaspoon black pepper
Pinch of hot red pepper flakes

Preheat the oven to 170°C (325°F or Mark 3). Halve the aubergines lengthwise, place them cut side down on a greased baking sheet and bake for 40 minutes, or until soft. Meanwhile, in a medium-sized non-stick frying pan sauté the red pepper, onion and garlic in the oil over medium heat for about 15 minutes, or until soft; set aside. Scoop the cooked aubergine flesh into a large bowl and mash it with a fork. Add the sautéed vegetables, tofu, Edam cheese, 2 tablespoons of the Parmesan, all but 2 tablespoons of the breadcrumbs, the parsley, salt and spices, and stir well. Transfer the mixture to a 1 litre (2 pint) baking dish, sprinkle with the remaining breadcrumbs and Parmesan and bake at the same temperature for 30 minutes.   Makes 4 servings

CALORIES per serving	200
45% Carbohydrate	24 g
23% Protein	12 g
32% Fat	8 g
CALCIUM	288 mg
IRON	3 mg
SODIUM	368 mg

SALMON MOUSSE

This dish provides 30 per cent of the daily requirement of iron for women.

500 g (1 lb) canned red salmon,
    liquid reserved
7 g (¼ oz) powdered gelatine
2 large spring onions
150 g (5 oz) frozen broad beans,
    thawed
2 teaspoons tomato paste
2 teaspoons prepared
    horseradish
1 teaspoon green peppercorns

12.5 cl (4 fl oz) Greek yogurt
12.5 cl (4 fl oz) plain low-fat
    yogurt
4 tablespoons lemon juice
60 g (2 oz) Cos lettuce, shredded
60 g (2 oz) spinach leaves,
    shredded
250 g (8 oz) asparagus, blanched
350 g (12 oz) loaf wholemeal
    French bread, sliced

Place 4 tablespoons of the salmon liquid in a small bowl, sprinkle in the gelatine and set aside for 5 minutes. Drain the salmon and discard any skin and large pieces of bone. Bring 12.5 cl (4 fl oz) of water to the boil, add it to the gelatine mixture and stir until the gelatine dissolves completely.

    Grease a 1 litre (2 pint) mould and set aside. In a food processor or blender, process the spring onions until minced. Add the salmon (including any small bones), the beans, tomato paste, horseradish and peppercorns, and process for about 1 minute, or until smooth. Add the gelatine mixture, yogurts and lemon juice and process just until combined, scraping down the container with a rubber spatula as necessary. Pour the mixture into the prepared mould and refrigerate for about 4 hours, or until the mousse is set.

    To unmould the mousse, invert the mould on a platter and briefly cover it with a tea towel wrung out in hot water. Surround the mousse with the lettuce, spinach and asparagus and serve with the bread.   Makes 6 servings

CALORIES per serving	375
44% Carbohydrate	41 g
27% Protein	26 g
29% Fat	12 g
CALCIUM	255 mg
IRON	3 mg
SODIUM	777 mg

BLACK-EYED PEA AND LENTIL SALAD

Pulses such as those in this salad contain all of the B vitamins except B$_{12}$.

75 g (2½ oz) dried black-eyed
    peas, soaked overnight
100 g (3½ oz) green lentils
½ teaspoon plus ⅛ teaspoon salt
125 g (4 oz) onion, finely chopped
4 tablespoons chopped parsley
1½ teaspoons lemon juice

1 teaspoon Dijon mustard
1 garlic clove, crushed
½ teaspoon dried thyme
⅛ teaspoon black pepper
1 teaspoon virgin olive oil
2 tablespoons low-sodium
    chicken stock

Place the lentils in a medium-sized saucepan with cold water to cover by 5 cm (2 inches). Bring to the boil over medium heat. Cover and simmer on low heat for 15 minutes. Drain the peas, add them to the pan and simmer for 45 minutes, or until the peas and lentils are tender, adding more water if needed. At the end of cooking, stir in ½ teaspoon of the salt.

    Drain the peas and lentils and transfer them to a medium-sized bowl. Stir in the onion and parsley. For the dressing, whisk together the lemon juice, mustard, garlic, thyme, pepper and the remaining salt in a small bowl. Slowly whisk in the oil in a thin stream, then add the stock, whisking constantly. Pour the dressing over the warm peas and lentils and toss well.   Makes 6 servings

CALORIES per serving	115
66% Carbohydrate	20 g
25% Protein	7 g
9% Fat	1 g
CALCIUM	35 mg
IRON	2 mg
SODIUM	268 mg

PENNE AND VEGETABLE SALAD

This dish provides iron and more than 100 per cent of your daily requirement of vitamin C, which helps your body absorb the iron.

CALORIES per serving	240
65% Carbohydrate	40 g
16% Protein	10 g
19% Fat	5 g
CALCIUM	95 mg
IRON	4 mg
SODIUM	284 mg

175 g (6 oz) asparagus, trimmed and cut into 2.5 cm (1 inch) pieces

125 g (4 oz) French beans, trimmed and cut into 2.5 cm (1 inch) pieces

600 g (1¼ lb) broccoli florets

125 g (4 oz) Swiss chard, trimmed and coarsely chopped

1 bunch watercress, trimmed and coarsely chopped

1 bunch rocket, trimmed and coarsely chopped

250 g (8 oz) penne

125 g (4 oz) spring onions, coarsely chopped

150 g (5 oz) frozen peas, thawed

125 g (4 oz) sweet red pepper, coarsely diced

4 tablespoons red wine vinegar, preferably balsamic

2 tablespoons olive oil, preferably extra-virgin

½ teaspoon hot red pepper flakes, or to taste

½ teaspoon salt

Bring a large pan of water to the boil. Blanch the asparagus, beans and broccoli together in the boiling water for 3 minutes. Reserving the boiling water, use a slotted spoon to transfer the blanched vegetables to a colander; cool the vegetables under cold water, drain them and transfer them to a large bowl. Blanch the chard, watercress and rocket together for 1 minute; drain them in a colander, cool them under cold water and drain again. Add the blanched greens to the bowl.

Refill the pan and bring the water to the boil. Cook the pasta according to the package directions until *al dente*; drain, rinse well and drain again. Add the pasta to the blanched vegetables, then add the remaining ingredients and toss well. Serve at room temperature or chilled.   Makes 6 servings

Penne and Vegetable Salad

BORSCHT

Vitamin B$_{12}$, found in chicken gizzards, is necessary for the production of red blood cells. This vitamin is present only in foods from animal sources.

1 tablespoon groundnut oil
350 g (12 oz) onions, coarsely chopped
100 g (3½ oz) celery, diced
5 chicken gizzards (125 g/4 oz), sliced 5 mm (¼ inch) thick
6 medium-sized beetroots, peeled and coarsely grated
25 cl (8 fl oz) low-sodium chicken stock
4 potatoes (about 600 g/1¼ lb total weight), peeled
2 tablespoons chopped fresh dill
1 teaspoon salt
¼ teaspoon black pepper
4 tablespoons soured cream

Heat the oil in a medium-sized saucepan over medium heat. Stir in the onion, celery and chicken gizzards, and sauté, stirring occasionally, for 10 minutes, or until the vegetables are soft. Stir in the beetroot and stock and bring to the boil. Reduce the heat to low, cover and simmer for 1 hour, or until the gizzards are tender. Meanwhile, place the potatoes in a large saucepan with cold water to cover, bring to the boil and cook for about 30 minutes, or until the potatoes are fork-tender; drain and set aside.

Add the dill, salt and pepper to the borscht and simmer for another 5 minutes. Place a potato in each of four bowls. Ladle the borscht into the bowls and garnish each serving with a tablespoon of soured cream.   Makes 4 servings

CALORIES per serving	270
48% Carbohydrate	27 g
20% Protein	11 g
32% Fat	8 g
CALCIUM	91 mg
IRON	4 mg
SODIUM	715 mg

MARINATED MUSHROOM-CAULIFLOWER SALAD

Besides being rich in B vitamins, this salad provides a fairly high level of beta carotene, a substance your body converts into vitamin A.

4 tablespoons white vinegar
4 tablespoons white wine or apple juice
2 teaspoons virgin olive oil
1 tablespoon brown sugar
1 garlic clove, crushed
½ teaspoon caraway seeds
¼ teaspoon cracked black peppercorns
¼ teaspoon salt
¼ teaspoon dried tarragon
300 g (10 oz) cauliflower florets
175 g (6 oz) small button mushrooms, trimmed
60 g (2 oz) spring onion greens, sliced
75 g (2½ oz) sweet red pepper, coarsely diced

For the marinade, combine the vinegar, wine, oil, sugar, garlic, caraway seeds, peppercorns, salt and tarragon in a large bowl or food-storage container; set aside. Bring 2 litres (3½ pints) of water to the boil in a large saucepan. Add the cauliflower, return the water to the boil and cook for 8 minutes. Using a slotted spoon, transfer the cauliflower to the marinade and toss to coat. Blanch the mushrooms in the boiling water for 1 minute; drain and add to the marinade. Add the spring onion greens and red pepper and toss to coat. Cover the bowl and refrigerate for at least 6 hours, or overnight.   Makes 4 servings

CALORIES per serving	85
59% Carbohydrate	14 g
15% Protein	4 g
26% Fat	3 g
CALCIUM	43 mg
IRON	2 mg
SODIUM	158 mg

Note: this salad will keep for up to five days in the refrigerator.

Stir-Fried Chicken and Vegetables

Dinner

STIR-FRIED CHICKEN AND VEGETABLES

The brown rice included in this dish contains more fibre and vitamin E than is found in polished white rice.

250 g (8 oz) brown rice
1 tablespoon plus 1 teaspoon
   sesame oil
350 g (12 oz) broccoli florets
175 g (6 oz) parsnips, cut into
   5 cm (2 inch) strips
1 medium-sized onion, sliced
½ sweet red pepper, cut into
   5 mm (¼ inch) strips
1½ teaspoons grated fresh
   ginger root
1½ teaspoons crushed garlic
1 teaspoon hot red pepper flakes

300 g (10 oz) skinless, boneless
   chicken breast, cut crosswise
   into 5 cm by 5 mm (2 by ¼ inch)
   thick strips
250 g (8 oz) spinach leaves
150 g (5 oz) fresh shiitake
   mushrooms, trimmed and sliced
30 g (1 oz) roasted cashew nuts
2 tablespoons Japanese rice-wine
   vinegar
1½ teaspoons low-sodium
   soy sauce
¼ teaspoon salt

Bring 80 cl (28 fl oz) of water to the boil in a medium-sized saucepan. Stir in the rice, cover, reduce the heat to low and cook for 40 minutes, or until the rice is tender and all of the water is absorbed; remove from the heat and set the pan aside.

In a large frying pan or wok, heat 1 tablespoon of the oil over high heat until rippling. Add the broccoli, parsnips, onion and sweet red pepper, and stir fry for 2 minutes, then add the ginger, garlic and red pepper flakes and stir fry for

CALORIES per serving	475
56% Carbohydrate	68 g
23% Protein	28 g
21% Fat	11 g
CALCIUM	152 mg
IRON	5 mg
SODIUM	339 mg

another 2 minutes. Using a slotted spoon, transfer the vegetables to a large bowl; set aside. Add the remaining oil to the wok or frying pan. Add the chicken and stir fry for 1½ minutes, separating the pieces. Return the cooked vegetables to the pan and add the spinach, mushrooms and cashews. Add the vinegar, soy sauce and salt, and stir fry for 2 minutes, or until the mushrooms are just cooked and the spinach is wilted. Divide the rice among four plates and spoon the chicken and vegetables on top.   Makes 4 servings

Note: shiitake mushrooms are available in some supermarkets. Use fresh white button mushrooms if shiitake are not available.

SWEETBREADS WITH SWEET POTATOES

Although sweetbreads are high in B vitamins and iron, they also contain a fair amount of cholesterol. Here the cholesterol per serving is kept low by using small portions of sweetbreads and lots of vegetables.

300 g (10 oz) calf's sweetbreads	**17.5 cl (6 fl oz) low-sodium beef stock**
½ small lemon	
500 g (1 lb) orange-fleshed sweet potatoes	**175 g (6 oz) mushrooms, sliced**
	8 stoned prunes, halved
2 teaspoons virgin olive oil	**Black pepper**
2 teaspoons cornflour	**4 tablespoons thinly sliced spring onions**
2 tablespoons medium-dry sherry	

Place the sweetbreads in a bowl with cold water to cover and place in the refrigerator to soak for 2 to 3 hours, changing the water once. Drain and rinse the sweetbreads and place them in a large non-reactive saucepan with cold water to cover. Add the lemon half, bring to the boil over medium-low heat and simmer for 5 minutes. Drain and rinse the sweetbreads and peel off the tough outer skin. Place the sweetbreads on a plate, place another plate on top and weight it with a heavy weight. Refrigerate for at least 4 hours, or overnight. (This firms the sweetbreads so they do not fall apart during cooking.)

Bring a large saucepan of water to the boil. Meanwhile, scrub the sweet potatoes. Cook the potatoes in the boiling water for about 35 minutes, or until tender. Meanwhile, preheat the oven to 130°C (250°F or Mark ½). Wrap the cooked potatoes in foil and place them in the oven to keep warm.

Slice the sweetbreads lengthwise into 5 mm (¼ inch) thick slices. Heat 1 teaspoon of oil in a large non-stick frying pan over medium heat. Sauté half of the sweetbreads for 2 minutes, or until golden-brown; transfer to an ovenproof platter. Add the remaining oil to the pan, cook the remaining sweetbreads and add them to the platter. Drain any accumulated juices from the platter into the frying pan, cover the platter with foil and place it in the oven to keep warm.

For the sauce, dissolve the cornflour in the sherry in a small bowl; set aside. Add the stock, mushrooms, prunes and black pepper to taste to the frying pan, bring to the boil over medium heat and cook for 5 minutes. Add the cornflour mixture and spring onions to the sauce and cook for another 2 minutes. Meanwhile, cut the sweet potatoes lengthwise into 5 mm (¼ inch) thick slices. Arrange alternating slices of potato and sweetbread on each of four plates and pour some of the sauce over each serving.   Makes 4 servings

CALORIES per serving	235
59% Carbohydrate	36 g
25% Protein	15 g
16% Fat	4 g
CALCIUM	48 mg
IRON	3 mg
SODIUM	83 mg

OYSTER STEW

Oysters contain substantial amounts of niacin, which is necessary for the synthesis of protein in your skin.

1 tablespoon safflower oil
3 tablespoons plain flour
50 cl (16 fl oz) skimmed milk
350 g (12 oz) potatoes, diced
25 cl (8 fl oz) low-sodium chicken
   stock
165 g (5½ oz) carrots, grated
125 g (4 oz) each sweet red and
   yellow pepper, coarsely diced
75 g (2½ oz) mushroom caps,
   sliced

4 tablespoons thinly sliced spring
   onions
4 tablespoons chopped shallots
12 small fresh oysters, shelled,
   with their liquor reserved
2 tablespoons chopped parsley
1 teaspoon Worcester sauce
1 teaspoon grated lemon rind
½ teaspoon salt
Dash of Tabasco sauce
75 g (2½ oz) spinach leaves,
   coarsely chopped

Heat the oil in a medium-sized heavy saucepan over medium heat. Add the flour and cook, stirring, for 3 minutes (the mixture should be dry but not browned). Slowly add the milk, one third at a time, whisking constantly until smooth. Add the potatoes and 12.5 cl (4 fl oz) of the stock, reduce the heat to low and cook for about 20 minutes, or until the potatoes are tender.

Meanwhile, in a medium-sized frying pan over medium heat, cook the carrots, sweet peppers, mushrooms, onions and shallots in the remaining stock for about 5 minutes, or until the vegetables are slightly wilted. Add the oysters and their liquor and cook until the oysters' edges are ruffled and the oysters are firm. Add the contents of the frying pan to the saucepan. Add the parsley, Worcester sauce, lemon rind, salt and Tabasco sauce, and stir to combine. Add the spinach, stir to combine and serve immediately.   Makes 4 servings

CALORIES per serving	230
63% Carbohydrate	37 g
19% Protein	11 g
18% Fat	5 g
CALCIUM	220 mg
IRON	5 mg
SODIUM	426 mg

BOSTON BAKED BEANS

A serving of this dish provides 100 per cent of the daily iron requirement for women.

500 g (1 lb) dried haricot beans
250 g (8 oz) onion, finely chopped
175 g (6 oz) molasses
4 tablespoons pure maple syrup
2 teaspoons dry mustard
1 teaspoon tomato paste

1 rasher bacon
250 g (8 oz) boneless pork loin,
   trimmed of fat
steamed brown bread (recipe
   follows)

Rinse the beans in cold water. Place them in a bowl with 1 litre (2 pints) of cold water and set aside to soak overnight. Or, to quick-soak, place the beans and water in a medium-sized saucepan, bring to the boil and simmer the beans for 2 minutes. Cover and set aside for 2 hours.

Pour off the soaking water, add 1 litre (2 pints) of fresh water and bring it barely to a simmer over low heat. Cook, covered, for 1¼ to 1½ hours, or until

CALORIES per serving with brown bread	755
69% Carbohydrate	134 g
20% Protein	37 g
11% Fat	10 g
CALCIUM	589 mg
IRON	18 mg
SODIUM	305 mg

the beans are tender. Do not boil the beans rapidly or they will split and break. Preheat the oven to 150°C (300°F or Mark 2). Drain the beans, reserving the liquid, and transfer them to a 2 litre (3½ pint) ovenproof casserole with a cover. (A heatproof plate can be used to cover a round casserole.) In a medium-sized bowl stir together the onion, molasses, maple syrup, mustard and tomato paste. Pour the mixture over the beans and toss gently with a rubber spatula to combine. Bury the bacon in the beans, cover the casserole tightly with foil and place the cover on it. Bake the beans for 2 hours, stirring about every 45 minutes. Add some of the reserved cooking liquid as necessary to keep the beans moist. Add the pork, pushing it down into the beans, and bake the beans for another 2 hours. Serve the pork and beans with steamed brown bread. Makes 4 servings

STEAMED BROWN BREAD

Leftover brown bread (the recipe yields three loaves) makes a good high-carbohydrate snack before you exercise. Because of its low fat content, the bread can be digested quickly and is less likely than rich pastries to upset your stomach during a workout.

75 g (2½ oz) raisins
60 g (2 oz) wholemeal flour
25 cl (8 fl oz) semi-skimmed milk
175 g (6 oz) molasses
4 tablespoons honey

1 tablespoon white vinegar
1 teaspoon grated orange rind
90 g (3 oz) cornmeal
45 g (1½ oz) rye flour
2 teaspoons bicarbonate of soda

Preheat the oven to 150°C (300°F or Mark 2). Lightly grease three small loaf tins or pudding basins. Place the raisins in a small bowl, add boiling water to cover and set aside to soak for 15 minutes; drain and pat dry. Toss the raisins with 1 tablespoon of the wholemeal flour; set aside.

In a medium-sized bowl, whisk together the milk, molasses, honey, vinegar and orange rind; set aside. In a large bowl, combine the remaining wholemeal flour, the cornmeal, rye flour and bicarbonate of soda, and make a well in the centre. Pour in the milk mixture and stir to moisten the dry ingredients, then mix the batter until smooth. Stir in the raisins. Ladle the batter into the tins, filling them about two thirds full. Cover each tin with a double thickness of foil, pressing it round the rim to seal it, and secure it with string or tape. Place the tins in a large casserole and add boiling water to a depth of 5 cm (2 inches). Cover the casserole with its lid or with foil and bake the bread for 3 hours.

Run a knife round the edges of the tins to loosen the bread, then place the loaves on a baking sheet and bake them for about 10 minutes, or until the crust is dried. Makes three 275 g (9 oz) loaves; each loaf is 4 servings

Note: the bread can also be steamed on top of the stove. Place a wire rack or trivet in the bottom of a large saucepan, stand the tins on the rack, add 5 cm (2 inches) of boiling water and cover tightly. Cook over low heat for 3 hours, adding boiling water if necessary to maintain the level in the tin. This bread freezes well. You can toast it for breakfast, spread it with cottage cheese for sandwiches or serve it with fruit salad or yogurt for dessert.

CALORIES per ¼ loaf	145
87% Carbohydrate	32 g
7% Protein	3 g
6% Fat	1 g
CALCIUM	125 mg
IRON	3 mg
SODIUM	162 mg

Snacks

FRUITY OATMEAL BISCUITS

The sesame seeds in these biscuits contain thiamine, niacin and vitamin B_6 as well as magnesium, a mineral essential for muscle contraction.

CALORIES per biscuit	65		
52% Carbohydrate	9 g		
10% Protein	2 g		
38% Fat	3 g		
CALCIUM	23 mg		
IRON	1 mg		
SODIUM	53 mg		

125 g (4 oz) rolled oats
60 g (2 oz) wholemeal flour
45 g (1½ oz) toasted wheat germ
60 g (2 oz) sesame seeds
75 g (2½ oz) currants
45 g (1½ oz) dates, chopped
1 teaspoon baking powder

½ teaspoon salt
60 g (2 oz) polyunsaturated
  margarine
100 g (3½ oz) brown sugar
1 large egg
1 teaspoon pure vanilla extract
1 teaspoon grated lemon rind

Preheat the oven to 190°C (375°F or Mark 5). In a medium-sized bowl, combine the oats, flour, wheat germ, sesame seeds, currants, dates, baking powder and salt, and stir until well mixed. In a large bowl, cream together the margarine and sugar. Add the egg and mix well. Add the vanilla extract and lemon rind and mix well. Add the dry ingredients and mix well. If the dough is too

Golden Trail Mix and
Fruity Oatmeal Biscuits

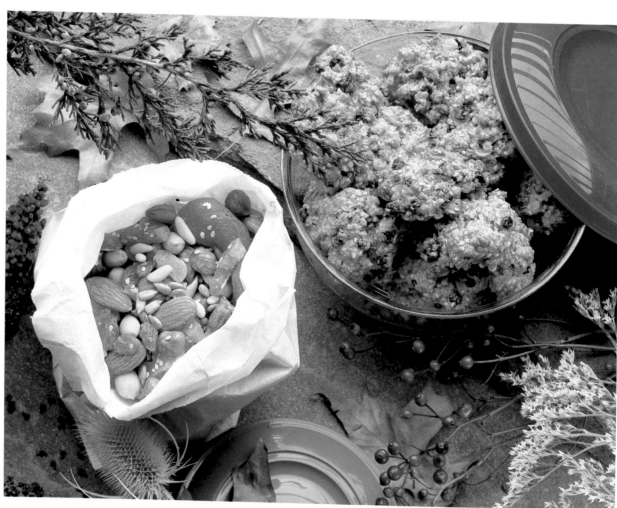

dry to drop from the spoon, add 1 or 2 tablespoons of water.

Drop spoonfuls of the dough on to non-stick baking sheets and flatten slightly. (The biscuits can be placed fairly close together since the dough does not spread very much.) Bake for 10 to 12 minutes, or until the biscuits are golden and their edges slightly browned. Cool the biscuits for 3 minutes on the baking sheets, then, using a spatula, carefully transfer them to racks to cool completely. Repeat with the remaining dough.   Makes 3 dozen biscuits

GOLDEN TRAIL MIX

A fruit-and-nut snack like this one, made without oil or sugar, contains less fat and more fibre than most muesli bars.

325 g (11 oz) sultanas

250 g (8 oz) unsulphured dried apricots

250 g (8 oz) each dried peaches and dried pears, cut into thin strips

90 g (3 oz) shelled peanuts

100 g (3½ oz) shelled unblanched almonds

100 g (3½ oz) crystallized ginger, cut into thin strips

60 g (2 oz) shelled hazelnuts

75 g (2½ oz) hulled sunflower seeds

25 g (¾ oz) pine-nuts

2 tablespoons sesame seeds

CALORIES per 30 g (1 oz)	150
61% Carbohydrate	25 g
9% Protein	4 g
30% Fat	6 g
CALCIUM	37 mg
IRON	2 mg
SODIUM	5 mg

Combine all of the ingredients in a large bowl and toss well. Refrigerate the trail mix in a tightly closed jar or polythene bag.   Makes about 1.3 kg (2 ¾ lb)

WALNUT FRUIT LOG

Both the wheat germ and the raisins in this recipe contain vitamin B$_6$, which is vital to the functioning of your immune system.

75 g (2½ oz) raisins

60 g (2 oz) unsulphured dried apricots

45 g (1½ oz) wheat germ

30 g (1 oz) shelled walnuts

1 teaspoon rum

Place all of the ingredients in a food processor or blender and process for 30 to 45 seconds, or until the texture resembles coarse crumbs. Scrape the mixture on to a sheet of foil and form it into a compact 15 by 4 cm (6 by 1½ inch) log. Wrap the log in a second sheet of foil and refrigerate overnight. (The flavour will improve with several days of refrigeration.) To serve, cut the fruit log into 12 slices.   Makes 12 servings

CALORIES per slice	65
62% Carbohydrate	11 g
12% Protein	2 g
26% Fat	2 g
CALCIUM	10 mg
IRON	1 mg
SODIUM	2 mg

Note: if you prefer, or if the fruit log is being served to children, substitute pure vanilla extract for the rum.

BUCKWHEAT-MUSHROOM PÂTÉ

Whole grains such as buckwheat groats (kasha) are an important source of dietary riboflavin. Studies show that women who are on weight-loss diets often do not consume enough riboflavin.

200 g (7 oz) buckwheat groats (kasha), medium grain
1 tablespoon plus 1 teaspoon groundnut oil
2 medium-sized whole carrots plus 125 g (4 oz) grated carrots
175 g (6 oz) mushrooms, thinly sliced
250 g (8 oz) onions, finely chopped

250 g (8 oz) whole spinach leaves, washed but not dried
4 tablespoons wheat germ
4 tablespoons Dijon mustard
4 large egg whites
1 teaspoon salt
½ teaspoon dried rosemary, crushed
½ teaspoon dried thyme, crumbled
¼ teaspoon black pepper

Bring 50 cl (16 fl oz) of water to the boil in a small saucepan. Stir in the kasha, reduce the heat to low, cover and simmer for 8 to 10 minutes, or until the kasha is fluffy and the water is absorbed; set aside, covered. Brush a 22 by 10 cm (9 by 4 inch) glass loaf dish with 1 teaspoon of the oil; set aside.

Half fill a large saucepan with water. Add the whole carrots, bring to a simmer and cook the carrots for 20 minutes, or until tender when pierced with a fork; drain and cool under cold water. Heat the remaining oil in a large non-stick frying pan over medium heat. Stir in the mushrooms, onions and grated carrots, cover and cook for about 5 minutes, or until the mushrooms release their liquid. Uncover the pan, reduce the heat to low and cook, stirring, for about 10 minutes, or until the vegetables are soft and all the liquid has evaporated; transfer to a large bowl and set aside.

Wipe out the frying pan with paper towels. Place the spinach in the pan, cover and steam over low heat for about 3 minutes, or just until the leaves are wilted; set aside.

Preheat the oven to 180°C (350°F or Mark 4). Using a fork, break up the kasha and stir it into the vegetable mixture. Add the wheat germ, 1 tablespoon of the mustard, the egg whites, salt, rosemary, thyme and pepper, and stir until well blended.

Line the loaf dish with the spinach leaves, overlapping them and leaving a 5 cm (2 inch) overhang round the top. Pack half of the kasha mixture into the dish, then lay the whole carrots lengthwise on top, 2.5 cm (1 inch) apart. Pack in the remaining kasha mixture and fold the overlapping spinach leaves over the top. Cover the pâté with foil, prick the foil in several places with a fork and place the loaf dish in a large roasting tin. Add 1 cm (½ inch) of hot water to the roasting tin and bake the pâté for 1½ hours.

When the pâté is done, cool the tin on a rack for 30 minutes, then refrigerate it overnight. Turn the pâté out on to a platter and use a sharp knife to cut it into 16 slices. Serve the remaining mustard with the pâté. Makes 16 servings

CALORIES per slice	60
57% Carbohydrate	9 g
18% Protein	3 g
25% Fat	2 g
CALCIUM	34 mg
IRON	1 mg
SODIUM	280 mg

CURRIED CHICK-PEA DIP WITH VEGETABLES

This recipe supplies 20 per cent of the RDA of iron for women and more than 75 per cent of your body's daily need for vitamin C.

CALORIES per serving	135
47% Carbohydrate	18 g
20% Protein	8 g
33% Fat	6 g
CALCIUM	118 mg
IRON	2 mg
SODIUM	147 mg

1 garlic clove, blanched and peeled (see page 127)

1 tablespoon chopped spring onion

150 g (5 oz) canned chick-peas, rinsed and drained

125 g (4 oz) ricotta cheese

2 teaspoons curry powder

½ teaspoon brown sugar

¼ teaspoon Worcester sauce

2 dashes Tabasco sauce

12.5 cl (4 fl oz) Greek yogurt

90 g (3 oz) cooked spinach, coarsely chopped

125 g (4 oz) mushrooms, trimmed

90 g (3 oz) mange-tout, blanched

8 asparagus spears, blanched

250 g (8 oz) broccoli florets, blanched

125 g (4 oz) yellow or green courgettes, cut into 7.5 cm (3 inch) sticks

1 orange-fleshed sweet potato, thinly sliced

Process the garlic and spring onion in a food processor or blender until well chopped. Add the chick-peas, ricotta, curry powder, sugar, Worcester sauce and Tabasco sauce, and process for about 30 seconds, or until smooth. Add the yogurt and spinach and process just until combined. Transfer to a bowl and serve with the vegetables as dippers.   Makes 6 servings

Curried Chick-Pea Dip with Vegetables

CALORIES per pretzel	170
78% Carbohydrate	34 g
13% Protein	6 g
9% Fat	2 g
CALCIUM	25 mg
IRON	2 mg
SODIUM	247 mg

WHEAT-BERRY PRETZELS

Yeast, such as the dried yeast used in these pretzels, is the richest naturally occurring source of riboflavin.

60 g (2 oz) wheat berries	**75 g (2½ oz) rye flour**
7 g (¼ oz) dried yeast	**¾ teaspoon salt**
1 tablespoon plus ¼ teaspoon sugar	**3 tablespoons bicarbonate of soda**
225 g (7½ oz) bread flour	**2 tablespoons sesame seeds**
125 g (4 oz) wholemeal flour	**2 tablespoons Dijon mustard**

Soak the wheat berries overnight in hot water to cover. Alternatively simmer the berries in 25 cl (8 fl oz) of water for 10 minutes. Place 6 tablespoons of warm water in a small bowl, stir in the yeast and ¼ teaspoon of the sugar and set aside for about 5 minutes, or until foamy. In a large bowl, combine half of the bread flour with the wholemeal and rye flours and the salt. Make a well in the centre, pour in the yeast mixture and 25 cl (8 fl oz) of warm water, and stir. Stir in half of the remaining bread flour, or as much as necessary to form a soft dough. Knead the dough on a floured board, working in the remaining flour, for about 10 minutes, or until smooth and elastic.

Grease a large bowl, place the dough in it and set it aside to rise in a warm place for about 2 hours, or until doubled in bulk. Meanwhile, drain the wheat berries and pat them dry.

Knock back the risen dough and knead in the wheat berries. Divide the dough into 12 equal pieces. Roll each piece into a 45 cm (18 inch) length, tapering the ends, then twist it into a pretzel shape and place it on a greased baking sheet. Let the dough rise again for about 40 minutes, or until the pretzels have almost doubled in bulk.

Preheat the oven to 220°C (425°F or Mark 7). Bring 1 litre (2 pints) of water, the bicarbonate of soda and the remaining sugar to a simmer in a large non-reactive frying pan. Place three pretzels in the water and cook for 1 minute, turning them after 30 seconds. Place the pretzels on a rack to drain for 10 minutes, then place them twisted side up on the baking sheets and sprinkle with sesame seeds. Repeat with the remaining pretzels, then bake for 15 minutes, or until browned and crisp. Cool the pretzels briefly on racks and serve them warm with the mustard. Makes 12 pretzels

CALORIES per pop	120
60% Carbohydrate	20 g
15% Protein	5 g
25% Fat	4 g
CALCIUM	8 mg
IRON	1 mg
SODIUM	26 mg

FROZEN BANANA POPS

The wheat germ used here has substantial quantities of vitamin B_6, the peanuts supply niacin and the banana is rich in potassium, giving this frozen treat a distinct nutritional advantage over an ice cream.

1 tablespoon finely chopped unsalted peanuts	**1 medium-sized ripe banana, peeled**
3 tablespoons toasted wheat germ	

Mix the peanuts and wheat germ on a plate. Cut the banana in half crosswise, dip each half in water and then roll it in the wheat germ mixture. Insert a wooden ice lolly stick into the cut end of each half, wrap in foil and freeze the pops for 3 to 4 hours, or until firm. Makes 2 banana pops

Beverages

PINEAPPLE-BERRY DRINK

Brewer's yeast is an excellent source of most of the B vitamins as well as trace minerals. While it has a strong taste, it becomes more palatable when mixed with other flavourful ingredients, as in this drink.

35 cl (12 fl oz) pineapple juice

60 g (2 oz) frozen raspberries

75 g (2½ oz) frozen strawberries

2 teaspoons brewer's yeast

Place all of the ingredients in a blender and process until smooth. Pour the drink into two glasses and serve immediately.

Makes 2 servings

CALORIES per serving	135
92% Carbohydrate	32 g
6% Protein	2 g
2% Fat	0.3 g
CALCIUM	39 mg
IRON	1 mg
SODIUM	6 mg

LEMON BARLEY-WATER CONCENTRATE

Soft drinks make poor fluid replacement beverages after exercise because their high sugar content slows your body's water absorption. This tangy drink base has no refined sugar, so the water in it is absorbed quickly.

100 g (3½ oz) pearl barley

12.5 cl (4 fl oz) lemon juice

Combine the barley with 1.5 litres (2½ pints) of water in a medium-sized saucepan and bring to a slow boil over medium heat. Skim the foam from the surface. Reduce the heat to low and simmer for 1 hour, skimming occasionally. Add 75 cl (1¼ pints) of water and simmer for another 30 minutes. Add 25 cl (8 fl oz) of water, then strain the mixture through a medium sieve placed over a bowl, pressing out all the liquid. Discard the barley. Stir in the lemon juice, let the mixture cool to room temperature, then transfer the concentrate to a bottle or jar, cover and refrigerate until chilled. It will keep for up to 2 weeks in the refrigerator.

For a lemon barley-water fizz, place a mint sprig in a tall glass and add 12.5 cl (4 fl oz) of the prepared concentrate; stir to crush the mint. Let stand for about 5 minutes, then stir in 25 cl (8 fl oz) of soda or mineral water. Serve immediately.

Makes 8 servings

CALORIES per serving	45
88% Carbohydrate	11 g
9% Protein	1 g
3% Fat	0.2 g
CALCIUM	4 mg
IRON	Trace
SODIUM	46 mg

NUT NOG

If possible, buy milk in opaque containers; in glass bottles, milk can lose up to 75 per cent of its riboflavin after only 3½ hours of exposure to light.

50 cl (16 fl oz) skimmed milk

1 tablespoon peanut butter

1 tablespoon honey

Pinch of cinnamon or nutmeg

Combine the milk, peanut butter and honey in a blender and process until thoroughly combined. For a cold drink, divide the mixture among three glasses and sprinkle with cinnamon. For a hot drink, pour the nut nog into a saucepan and heat over medium-low heat, stirring, just until warm.

Makes 3 servings

CALORIES per serving	100
48% Carbohydrate	13 g
27% Protein	7 g
25% Fat	3 g
CALCIUM	219 mg
IRON	Trace
SODIUM	105 mg

ACKNOWLEDGEMENTS

The Editors wish to thank Kate Cann and Norma MacMillan.

Index prepared by Ian Tucker.

PHOTOGRAPHY CREDITS

Cover: Julian Bajzert, London; pages 34-35: Steven Mays; pages 38-47: Mark Ledzian; pages 48-55: Steven Mays; pages 58-77, page 78: Gudrun Bergdahl/Vandystadt/Photo Researchers; page 78, inset: Gerard Vandystadt/Vandystadt/Photo Researchers; page 80, left: Roger Tully, right: Thought Technology, Ltd.; page 81: Roger Tully; page 83: Larry Dale Gordon/The Image Bank; pages 84-85: Hank Morgan/Rainbow; pages 86-87, 90-95: Steven Mays; pages 96-119, Ariel Skelley; pages 120-121, 124-141: Steven Mays.

ILLUSTRATION CREDITS

Page 8, illustration: David Flaherty; page 11, illustration: David Flaherty; page 12, illustration: David Flaherty; page 15, illustration: David Flaherty; page 18, illustration: David Flaherty; page 21, illustration: Brian Sisco; page 24, illustration: Brian Sisco; pages 28-29, illustration: Brian Sisco; page 31, illustration: Brian Sisco and Tammy Colichio; page 32, illustration, David Flaherty; page 57, illustration: Brian Sisco.

Typeset by A.J. Latham Limited,
Dunstable, Bedfordshire
Printed by GEA, Milan and bound by GEP,
Cremona, Italy

INDEX